The Antidepressant Sourcebook:

a user's guide for patients and families

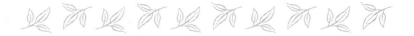

a user's guide for patients and families

The Antidepressant Sourcebook

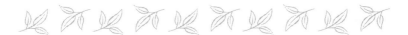

ANDREW L. MORRISON, M.D.

MAIN STREET BOOKS
DOUBLEDAY

New York   London   Toronto   Sydney   Auckland

A MAIN STREET BOOK
PUBLISHED BY DOUBLEDAY
a division of Random House, Inc.
1540 Broadway, New York, New York 10036

MAIN STREET BOOKS, DOUBLEDAY, and the portrayal of a
building with a tree are trademarks of Doubleday, a division of
Random House, Inc.

Book design by Ellen Cipriano

Library of Congress Cataloging-in-Publication Data Applied For

ISBN 0-385-49665-6

Printed in the United States of America

January 2000

1   3   5   7   9   10   8   6   4   2

First Edition

In memory of M.
This book is dedicated to those about to lose hope.
May it inspire them not to give up.

Portions of the proceeds of this book will be donated to NARSAD (the National Alliance for Research on Schizophrenia and Depression). NARSAD is a national, not-for-profit organization whose primary objective is to raise funds to find the causes, cures, better treatments, and prevention of the severe mental illnesses. It was founded more than ten years ago by family members and professionals who are convinced that a better future can be found through expanded brain research.

Acknowledgments

To my wife, Candy, I give most of my gratitude. Without her creativity, encouragement, editing skills, and tolerance of my peccadilloes, this book would never have become a reality.

Similarly, had I not had the support of Jonathan Cole, M.D., and John Greist, M.D., I doubt that this book would have happened. Dr. Greist's painstaking review of every page is immeasurably appreciated.

Several very good friends also helped with the manuscript, and I remain indebted to them for their helpful comments: Jack Adair, M.D., David Giles, M.D., Sarah Hofheinz, and Penny Stone. A specific thank-you must go to my close friend Jim Hunt, M.D. ("the Master"), who first taught me the fundamentals and art of prescribing psychiatric medicine. Thanks also to Mom and Dad for their unceasing encouragement, and to Toad Atwill, Lisa Havens, and Linda Hegeman for their assistance.

Laurie Casey, and especially Pam Barker, performed typing duties with nary an error, and in such a timely fashion that I simply couldn't have asked for more. Thanks particularly to wordsmith Rianne Keedy for the finishing touches.

I will be forever grateful to two special mentors, the late Drs. Clare Assue and Bill Fisher, who both embodied and taught what it takes to be a responsible psychiatrist. Thanks also to Jim Coles, Dick Darko, and Craig Pinkus for their advice, both legal and otherwise.

I am also quite grateful to Carol Ascherman, Ron Diersing, Susan Kanipe, Laura Klinestiver, and Scott Clark for their assistance, and for the cooperation of the following pharmaceutical companies (in alphabetical order): Bristol-Myers Squibb, Eli Lilly and Company, Forest, Glaxo Wellcome, Hoechst Marion Roussel, Merck, Novartis, Organon, Oxford, Parke-Davis, Pfizer, Sandoz, SmithKline Beecham, Solvay, and Wyeth-Ayerst.

Finally I'd like to especially thank Jennifer Griffin, my editor, her talented assistants, Katy Burns-Howard and Jay Crosby, and Main Street Books / Doubleday for being so easy to work with. I am extremely appreciative of their help in spreading the word about these wondrous antidepressant medications and for taking part in the battle against depression.

Contents

17. Alcohol, Caffeine, and Recreational Drugs, Part I 91

What to Expect

18. The Therapeutic Alliance, Part II: Working Together 99
19. Aesop's Tortoise 101
20. Which Antidepressant is "the Best"? Finding the Right Medicine 109
21. Finding the Right Dose 119
22. Know When to Take It 123
23. Blood Levels 128
24. Peaks and Valleys, Chunks of Time 131
25. When and If to Stop an Antidepressant 136
26. How to Stop an Antidepressant 146

Warnings

27. Unilateral Dose Adjustments 151
28. Alcohol, Caffeine, and Recreational Drugs, Part II 154
29. Interactions with Other Drugs and Food 159
30. What About Side Effects? 164
31. What About Surgery and Dental Procedures? 169
32. What About Pregnancy and Breast-Feeding? 171
33. Cause and Effect 179
34. Psychotherapy 186
35. The Significance of Others 189
36. Relapses and Recurrences 192
37. Prevention 194
38. Giving Up 197

APPENDIX A The Antidepressants 205
APPENDIX B Organizations You Should Contact 209
FURTHER READING 213
INDEX 277

Preface

IT WAS THE KIND OF day that people say depresses them. It was February 1972, and things outside looked stark and colorless. The monotonous gray shade of the sky seemed to pervade everything, and it did not change as the hours dragged on. "How ironic," I thought, as I stared at the barren tree I could see through the hospital window. It looked so depressing outside, yet inside I was jubilant, brimming with excitement about the future.

Just two years out of medical school, I was working in the psychiatry residency program that had been my first choice. I was learning more and more every day, and I loved it. Furthermore, I had a wife and a two-year-old son who seemed perfect. I had doubted if life could get any better, but my wife became pregnant again, and I was with her as she lay in labor. Maybe it *could* get better!

And it did. Her labor was long and hard, but the delivery went well and my wife and new baby were both healthy. I had a wonderful night's sleep and my joyous mood continued into the next morning. I laughed out loud at the on-air antics of a disc jockey while driving to work. Outside the car, it was still overcast and gray, like a Russian winter day, but inside I felt buoyant.

After arriving at the psychiatric hospital, I began turning my attention to my patients, one of whom had depression. I had been learning about depression for several years. I had read articles and books and had attended lectures, so I was pretty "book smart" about it. But early this morning, still effervescent inside, it was especially hard for me to fathom what depression must really feel like.

The patient with depression was named Mark. Mark was nineteen when his parents took him to their family physician because of their concern about his personality change. He just didn't seem to care about anything anymore. Previously sociable and a decent student, he had become quiet and withdrawn and had lost his work ethic. He slept a lot and never laughed like he used to. Mark admitted to his family physician that he seemed to have lost his interest in doing the things that he previously enjoyed, and, among other things, he wondered if everybody, including himself, would be better off if he were dead.

The family physician had examined Mark and performed the appropriate laboratory tests to rule out other illnesses, like hypothyroidism, that sometimes mimic depression. Mark's depression was diagnosed and treated appropriately for about a month but had not responded well to outpatient treatment. This continued depression and lack of response to treatment is what led to Mark's admission to the psychiatric hospital and is how Mark came to be under my care.

Mark and I had hit it off. We both enjoyed playing and watching basketball, and what was left of Mark's sense of humor was still engaging. We liked each other and had worked well together for over two months. Mark worked hard in psychotherapy and took his medicine as prescribed. As expected, there was definite improvement. So much so, in fact, that I had recommended a weekend furlough out of the hospital (a common practice back in 1972) in order to see how prepared Mark was for final discharge. He was due back that morning at eight o'clock.

By nine, Mark had not returned. A few hours later his family called to say they had found Mark's body in the garage. He had shot himself through the head. Adrenaline pumping and heart pounding, I made a beeline to the office of the professor who was supervising the case. I had had patients die before: of cancer, of heart disease, and of other things. But there was something different about this. It should not have happened, and I found myself sobbing. "Mark was better; I know he was better!" God, how I hurt inside.

Although I was initially wrapped up in my own pain and guilt, after a while I managed to shift my thinking to how much pain Mark's family was in. Then I thought of how much pain Mark must have been in, and I tried to imagine what Mark's pain felt like. For a few fleeting moments, I could feel its cold-blooded chill. It was evil and heartless, and it penetrated my gut. I will never forget it, and I swore to myself that I would always fight it with everything I had.

Now, more than twenty-five years later, it is comforting to know that we have made headway in the fight against depression. More and more people are learning that depression is a treatable medical illness and, even better, learning to recognize it. The causes of depression, and how to treat it more effectively, are now being researched with millions of dollars every year. Better and faster forms of psychotherapy—geared specifically for depression—are being developed. Ten to fifteen more antidepressants have been added to our treatment arsenal—medicines whose greater chemical accuracy and fewer side effects make them not just acceptable but eagerly sought after.

This book is about these antidepressant medications and should supply you with the basic, fundamental information you need to use them in the proper way. I hope it will help you in your fight against depression.

Foreword

I WAS INTRIGUED WHEN Dr. Morrison asked me to review this book. From time to time, I've thought of writing a similar book but have never done so. Now that I have read this book carefully, I'm delighted with it. It is as accurate as it is possible to be in a gradually changing field; I found no fact or suggestion that I wished to alter.

The book is very well written in clear, sensible—and sometimes mildly humorous—English. It is divided into thirty-eight chapters, well titled, so that it can be read easily in a few hours by any literate layperson, patient or relative. The book can be used as a reference work as well, to be consulted if questions or problems present themselves as someone considers, or takes part in, antidepressant therapy.

It distills very well the lessons Dr. Morrison has learned in his twenty-five years in the practice of psychiatry. He has read, listened, talked, and learned. From these experiences, he has written a highly useful book viewing antidepressant drug therapy from the patient's or family's vantage point—a valuable and highly sensible thing to do. He has done it very well.

Recent surveys of the outcomes of antidepressant drug treatments have clearly shown that many patients fail to benefit because they do not take the prescribed antidepressant for more than a few weeks. I suspect one of the major reasons this happens is a failure in communication between doctor and patient and between patient and doctor. Physicians in training or in practice will benefit from reading this book; it will help them work sensitively and sensibly with their patients. It will also help them handle their patients' questions, fears, doubts, and discouragements, and work toward a literally happy initial outcome and a long-term, relapse-free course.

As managed care and other forces work to shorten contacts between doctors and patients, books like this will help both patient and physician make optimum use of the times available.

JONATHAN O. COLE, M.D.
Professor of Psychiatry
Harvard Medical School
Senior Consultant
McLean Hospital
Belmont, Massachusetts

Introduction

THE GOAL OF THIS BOOK is to provide pragmatic and useful information to people who are taking, or contemplating taking, antidepressant medication, and for their families. If you are one of these people, please do not feel alone. In 1999, approximately 135 million prescriptions were filled in the United States for antidepressants.

There are more than twenty antidepressants on the market. Fortunately, they have enough in common that what is written here applies to all of them. They are discussed as a group, and you will find no favoritism or commercial bias within these pages.

Certain questions are always asked about the antidepressants. These are good, legitimate, commonsense questions, the same type of questions that patients and families ask about any medicine. This book answers these questions.

In addition to questions, patients and families will occasionally have unfounded fears and misconceptions, stemming from rumors and gossip about these medicines. This book will set the record straight and debunk the myths and fallacies about the antidepressants.

This book tells you what to expect when taking an antidepressant and, just as important, what *not* to expect. It addresses the issue of "chemical imbalances in the brain" and explains what the medicine can do and what it can't do. It also advises you on what to do and what not to do while taking an antidepressant.

Of major significance, it provides guidance on what to say to your doctor and on what you can do to promote a constructive working relationship with him or her. Then, by helping you manage your medicine as a team, it can shorten the time it takes to find the right medicine and the right dose for you. It also describes how to use the medication along with psychotherapy and the nonpharmacological components of treatment.

Additionally, the book gives pointers on specific subjects such as side effects, what to do if you forget a dose, planning a pregnancy, and so on. Furthermore, it provides vital information on how to collaborate with your doctor when it is time to address the inevitable issue of coming off the medicine.

When a patient is taking an antidepressant, these subjects will eventually be addressed by the doctor. Thousands of doctors, in many different languages, talk with their patients about this book's contents every day. But there is a great deal of ground to cover in just one (or even more than one) appointment, and rarely does a doctor have enough time to cover all these points in one sitting. Additionally, patients and families are often emotionally overwhelmed during the appointment and do not think to ask these questions, let alone accurately remember everything the doctor said. This book enables a patient and family to sit down and learn about the antidepressants when their frame of mind is relaxed and receptive. Moreover, the material can be read (and reread) at a comfortable pace, a pace that allows the brain to register and retain the information.

Patient anecdotes are scattered throughout the book to help make certain points and to give examples of important dos and don'ts. The examples are based on actual case histories, with the particulars changed to protect confidentiality. The use of anecdotes based on actual patients speaks to the fact that this book is about real people and it was written for real people—like yourself or your family member.

Interestingly, a significant percentage of the people who take antidepressants are not depressed. Depression is not the only condition treated by the antidepressants, and the information in this book is relevant to anyone taking an antidepressant—not just somebody with depression. For example, the FDA has approved the "on-label" use of certain antidepressants for treatment of panic disorder, obsessive-compulsive disorder, and bulimia nervosa, social phobia, and generalized anxiety disorder. Additionally, the antidepressants are prescribed "off-label" to treat pain, anxiety, attention-deficit/hyperactivity disorder, post-traumatic stress disorder, premenstrual dysphoric disorder, social phobia, and obsessive-compulsive-related disorders such as compulsive hair pulling, compulsive gambling, compulsive buying, sexual addictions, and kleptomania. Quite a mix!

Though this book supplies tips on how to work with your doctor to properly take an antidepressant, please note that it is no substitute for the doctor and is by no means intended to help people learn how to treat themselves. (To paraphrase a wise old saying, "The person who treats himself has a fool for a patient.") Quite the opposite is true: this book is meant to promote a positive relationship with your doctor and to facilitate your doctor's care. It is an adjunct to what the doctor says. If it results in better cooperation and teamwork between the patient, the patient's family, and the doctor, it has done its job.

It should be emphasized that this information is not just for patients—it is also for families and loved ones. The more family members and loved ones understand the antidepressants, the more they will be able to help and support the person taking the medicine. An ideal recovery involves the understanding and support of "significant others."

This book is a summary of what I think is the most important information for patients and families to know about these medicines. It is based on my experience as a psychiatrist, working more than fifty hours a week for over twenty-five years, treating patients with these medicines. Having primarily treated adults, I have limited the book's contents primarily to what is relevant to adults, though some of the principles apply to children and adolescents too. This, then, is my database: twenty-five years of reading, going to conferences, and talking with colleagues; twenty-five years of treating patients who have had the same questions, fears, myths, and misconceptions; twenty-five years of seeing what has worked and what has not worked. All of this, boiled down to the nitty-gritty, is what you'll find in the following pages.

The antidepressant medications can vastly improve the quality of life of people afflicted with certain psychiatric conditions and can even save lives. All too often, though, because patients and families do not know enough of the simple facts, these medicines are never taken, are taken incorrectly, or are stopped too soon. Consequently, treatment success is not as good as it could be. It is tragic that there continues to be so much suffering, and even death, due to incomplete treatment or no treatment of these very treatable conditions.

The Antidepressant Sourcebook will help people get the most out of their medicine. It is my hope that it will make a difference for all of its readers.

The Basics

I

The Antidepressants

THE ANTIDEPRESSANTS ARE a group of prescription medicines used for the treatment of depression as well as other psychiatric and medical conditions. Man's attempts to treat these disorders date back thousands of years, when the first surgeons drilled holes in the skulls of their patients (who had no anesthesia!) in order to expel "the demons within." Over the centuries, other treatment regimens have included bloodletting, exorcism, voodoo, magic potions, dietary supplements, herbal elixirs, and other home remedies, but no treatment was proved to be truly effective until the latter half of the twentieth century. The legitimacy of the antidepressant medications has withstood the scrutiny of hundreds of rigorously controlled scientific studies, and it is further substantiated by the millions of people all over the world who have benefited from them.

How the antidepressants got their start is an interesting tale, similar to how other discoveries in the field of medicine occurred: from a combination of luck and keen observation. Remember, for example, Sir Alexander Fleming's observation of what happened after a bacterial culture in his laboratory was accidentally contaminated by a mold. This led to the discovery of penicillin and the explosion of research on the antibiotics. The story of the antidepressants is just as fascinating.

It all started in the 1950s. While researching a medicine, iproniazid, to treat tuberculosis, doctors noticed that some of the patients receiving this medicine experienced elevation of their mood (even though their tuberculosis didn't improve). Based on this astute observation, researchers changed course and began studying iproniazid as a possible treatment for depression. One road taken by researchers was to explore the interaction between iproniazid and a medicine called reserpine. Reserpine was used at that time to treat high blood pressure. The researchers were interested in it because one of its side effects was depression. Iproniazid, investigators discovered, reversed some of reserpine's effects, which confirmed the scientists' belief that they were onto something.

Also in the 1950s, a new medicine, imipramine, was being studied as a possible treatment for psychosis. Thorazine had just been discovered to have astonishing antipsychotic effects in people with schizophrenia, and imipramine was chemically similar to Thorazine. As it turned out, imipramine did not help the psychotic symptoms of people with schizophrenia, but it was noted to have some antidepressant effects. As was occurring with iproniazid, imipramine research then changed its course, and shortly thereafter, the first antidepressants were introduced. In the late 1950s, iproniazid and imipramine were released in the United States under the brand names Marsilid and Tofranil.

Efforts to solve the mystery of exactly how the antidepressants work also make an interesting tale. But before we get into that, let's take a quick course in Nerve Chemistry 101. The most important thing to remember is that it takes a chemical reaction for a nerve impulse, traveling along one nerve, to fire off a second nerve. Unlike the chemical reactions created in high school chemistry labs, which seem to take forever and often make students late to their next class, these reactions occur almost instantaneously. The miraculousness of this speed is matched only by the phenomenally small space in which these reactions occur. This space, the gap between the two nerves, is called a synapse. For the last fifty years, antidepressant research has focused more on these chemical reactions in the synapse than on anything else.

The first nerve releases chemicals into the synapse, and these chemicals stimulate receptors on the second nerve, firing off the second nerve and thereby transmitting the neural (nerve) impulse. Because they *transmit* the *neural* impulse, these chemicals are called *neurotransmitters*. The word "neurotransmitter" may be the most important word to know in the field of antidepressant research. However, don't forget that the neurotransmitters stimulate *receptors* on the second nerve. What happens at the receptor sites is now being investigated as much as the neurotransmitters themselves, so the word "receptor" is becoming equally important.

Now, back to the 1950s again. Scientists knew that reserpine lowered blood pressure via its action, in the circulatory system, on a class of chemicals called the catecholamines. Catecholamines, significantly, are also present in the brain. Perhaps, they theorized, it was reserpine's effect on the catecholamines in the *brain* that caused the side effect of depression. And since iproniazid could reverse the effect of reserpine, perhaps iproniazid's antidepressant effect was related to its effect on brain catecholamines. Early research results confirmed these suspicions: iproniazid did affect brain catecholamines, which, as it turned out, do function in the brain as neurotransmitters. Researchers also found another neurotransmitter—one called serotonin. But the early studies focused mainly on the catecholamines.

What became known as the catecholamine hypothesis postulated that the success of the antidepressants had something to do with their affecting (possibly increasing the level of) catecholamines in the synapse. Here is a simplified version of the theory: In a normal brain, without any antidepressant present, after the catecholamines do their job of stimulating the receptors in the synapse, a portion of the catecholamines is reabsorbed back into the first nerve again. This process is called reuptake. Additionally, another portion of the catecholamines is broken down by an enzyme—the first step in the journey to the kidneys and eventual elimination from the body. When an antidepressant is present, however, the reuptake and/or the breakdown process is inhibited, resulting in an increased level of catecholamines in the synapse.

Excitement grew as investigators conducted studies to test the hypothesis. Was there just a deficiency of neurotransmitters in the synapse in depressed people to begin with? Did the antidepressants then correct this deficiency, raising the neurotransmitters to a normal level, thereby "fixing" the depression? Unfortunately, this theory was too easy an answer and didn't pan out in reality. The results of the studies just didn't fit the hypothesis. In fact, as often happens in research, there were more questions raised than answers found. To this day, researchers are still unable to find a hypothesis that puts all the pieces of the puzzle together and explains everything.

Fortunately, though, while much of the early research attention was on the catecholamines, some resolute researchers doggedly pursued this other neurotransmitter called serotonin. By the 1980s, medications had been developed that affected primarily serotonin, not catecholamine, neurotransmission.

Still other investigators focused their efforts on the receptors on the second nerve. They found a variety of different receptors and learned that the brain, its jumbled mass of interconnected nerves, and the entire body all respond differently, depending on which receptors are stimulated more (or less) than others. Before long, the serotonin receptors they discovered numbered in the double digits.

Research reached new heights as the 1980s gave way to the 1990s. Invaluable advocacy groups helped protect indispensable government grants, which were annually threatened by budget trimmers. For the first time in history, pharmaceutical companies were making significant profits from antidepressant sales. Competition in the private sector intensified and accelerated the pace of research as these companies raced to find better medicines. Scientists began designing "designer drugs"—a far cry from the serendipitous discoveries of doctors researching tuberculosis, high blood pressure, and schizophrenia in the 1950s. Proactively, chemists altered the architecture and chemical properties of molecules in order to produce a desired effect on the neurotransmitters and receptors.

Despite the huge amount of time, energy, and money that went into new antidepressant research in the 1990s, many of the older medicines still remain on the market today. Just as penicillin continues to be a dependable weapon in our arsenal of antibiotics, so does Tofranil continue to be a reliable weapon in our antidepressant arsenal. Though iproniazid is now off the market, a dozen or so other antidepressants were introduced in the 1960s and 1970s. They, like Tofranil, have withstood the test of time, and continue to be reliable and effective antidepressants. They are the "old faithful" antidepressants.

The old faithful antidepressants, though, have a relatively broad, wide-spectrum effect on neurotransmitters and receptors (and the rest of the body as well). Therefore, they are more likely to have other consequences in the body besides the desired effects. These other consequences include sleepiness, dry mouth, constipation, weight gain, blurred vision, increased heart rate, and a drop in blood pressure (and therefore, lightheadedness or even fainting) upon standing.

Although all the searching in the 1980s and 1990s never found exactly how the antidepressants work, it did result in the birth of medicines called the new generation antidepressants. These medicines have a narrower, more focused effect on the neurotransmitters and receptors. Their "smart bomb" precision allows them to be just as effective as the old faithful antidepressants, but with fewer side effects on the rest of the body.

Currently, one of the new generation antidepressants is usually prescribed before an old faithful antidepressant, though sometimes a patient may need more of a broad-spectrum effect and an old faithful antidepressant will therefore be prescribed first. Prozac was the first new generation antidepressant in the United States. It was introduced in 1988 and primarily affects serotonin. Currently, about ten new generation antidepressants have received FDA approval and are available in the United States.

Tricyclics, MAOIs, and SSRIs

Often an antidepressant is identified as being a member of the tricyclic, MAOI, or SSRI class. Although this classification system is not entirely satisfying, nothing better has come along to replace it, so these terms have endured. The names tricyclic, MAOI, and SSRI stem from the chemical properties of the medicines in each respective category. Fortunately, though, you don't need a Ph.D. in chemistry to understand their evolution.

Let's start with the tricyclics. Imipramine, the first tricyclic, was initially studied as a drug for the treatment of psychosis. The reason it was being studied in the first place was that its chemical structure was similar to another drug, Thorazine, which had just been discovered to have strikingly beneficial effects on people with schizophrenia. The backbone of this Thorazine molecule consisted of three intertwined circular structures called benzene rings, and scientists were frantically investigating other molecules that also had this three-ringed structure. Imipramine had such a structure. In the two decades after imipramine's antidepressant effects were discovered, researchers found several other molecules that had both antidepressant properties and three benzene rings. Imipramine and its three-ringed descendants constitute the tricyclic class. They are named after their chemical anatomy, not after their chemical activity.

The MAOIs and the SSRIs, on the other hand, are named after their chemical activity, not their chemical structure. First, let's look at the MAOIs. MAOI is an abbreviation for "monoamine oxidase inhibitor." Remember how the effects of reserpine and iproniazid led investigators to study the catecholamines in the brain, and how a portion of the catecholamines are broken down by an enzyme? Iproniazid, studies showed, increased the level of catecholamines in the synapse by inhibiting the activity of this enzyme. This enzyme is called monoamine oxidase. Iproniazid thus became known as a monoamine oxidase inhibitor. Several other antidepressants have descended from iproniazid. They also inhibit this enzyme and are also called MAOIs.

The term SSRI stands for "selective serotonin reuptake inhibitor." The SSRIs are all newer antidepressants, rendering a relatively precise, focused effect on brain chemistry. They primarily affect the neurotransmitter serotonin, hence the first part of their name: selective serotonin. Like all antidepressants, their activity results in the buildup of neurotransmitters in the synapse, but they go about it in a different way than the MAOIs. Typically a portion of the neurotransmitters, after they stimulate the receptors on the second nerve, are reabsorbed back into the first nerve. The SSRIs inhibit this reabsorption process, giving rise to the last part of their name: reuptake inhibitors.

Identifying an antidepressant as a tricyclic, an MAOI, or an SSRI, although commonly done, can be confusing. The problem is that some of the antidepressants don't fit into any of these three categories. Some of the new generation antidepressants affect not only serotonin neurotransmission but also catecholamine neurotransmission: specifically, a neurotransmitter called norepinephrine. Additionally, some new generation antidepressants primarily affect norepinephrine and barely affect serotonin at all! Hence, some of the new generation antidepressants are not really selective *serotonin* reuptake inhibitors, but neither are they tricyclics or MAOIs. Furthermore, researchers are exploring entirely different types of neurotransmitters, such as the peptides, which include the neurokinins like Substance P. So the nomenclature is going to get even more confusing.

2

Depression

PATIENTS AND THEIR LOVED ONES rarely, if ever, recognize depression when it first hits. *Something* is wrong, and those affected *know* that something is wrong, but it is not identified as depression. They recognize that there is a "problem," but different aspects of that problem are perceived as more or less prominent, depending on the individual who is doing the perceiving. For example, one person may perceive himself as "being under a lot of stress right now." Another person may perceive herself as "going through a rough time with my . . ." (insert choice of specific stressor—significant other, finances, job, family member, or whatever). A third person may predominantly perceive himself as suffering from insomnia and fatigue. All three of these people may have clinical depression, but not recognize it for what it really is. Often it takes weeks or months before "the problem" is viewed from another angle and is recognized as depression.

On the contrary, a common cold or a heart attack is usually

recognized quickly. We experience the characteristic stuffy nose or pain in the chest and we immediately think, "Oh no, I'm getting a cold" or "Oh God, I wonder if I'm having a heart attack!" The symptoms of these disorders are universally known "red flags" that quickly lead us to identify the probable culprit.

But it doesn't work that way with depression, and, consequently, the affected person and the family try other means to fix "the problem" until something happens to turn on the lightbulb: "Hey, I wonder if this is depression."

Once the depression is recognized and diagnosed, it is time to learn about it. It should be noted that, for a significant other, learning about depression doesn't provide a total understanding of what it's really like to be depressed. Learning about depression can provide the significant other with an *intellectual* understanding of the illness, but that's not the same as being there. Indeed, there may be no words that can truly capture what it's like to be depressed. Consider this comparison: a man can learn and read about what it's like to have a baby, but until he gives birth himself, he won't know what it's really like. However, it should be emphasized that learning about depression can help immensely, while failure to do so can have disastrous consequences.

Whether you are the person afflicted with depression or a family member or a friend, it is comforting to know that "the problem" is a known entity, as opposed to something that nobody can do anything about and that nobody understands. It is reassuring to be able to make a little sense out of what's happened. And when it comes to treating the depression, understanding exactly what you are fighting makes you better prepared for battle.

Antidepressant medication, the subject of this book, is usually included in the treatment of depression. But before we start discussing the antidepressants, let's ensure that we have the same general understanding of what this thing called depression really is.

First, let's distinguish between the illness of depression and "normal" depression, because doesn't everybody get "depressed" from time to time? And if so, is everybody supposed to take an antidepressant from time to time?

Sure, everybody gets depressed at times, but there is a difference between the "normal" depressed *mood* that we all experience at one time or another (and for which we should not be medicated) and the *illness* depression. Unfortunately, the words "depression" and "depressed" are commonly used to refer to both conditions. These two words are thrown around loosely in everyday conversation, making it confusing and difficult to understand the difference between normal depressed moods and the illness depression. *The difference lies in the severity, the duration, and the other "signs and symptoms" that accompany the illness.*

Although the illness depression does not affect everybody in the same way—it has different aspects to it and may present itself in a variety of ways—a central feature is usually (but not always) a depressed, blue, sad mood, or at least a significant drop in the pleasure and enjoyment one is getting out of life. But with the illness depression, in contrast to "normal" depression, this mood disturbance is not mild or brief; it is there for weeks or more. It is there the majority of the time. It is there to the extent that it significantly interferes with one's life.

Furthermore, with the illness depression, other signs and symptoms occur along with the depressed mood. Only a minority of people with the illness depression have *all* these "associated signs and symptoms," but everybody with the illness depression has at least *some* of them. These associated signs and symptoms include sleep disturbance (increased or decreased sleep), appetite or weight disturbance (increased or decreased significantly), thinking difficulties (e.g., trouble with concentration, attention span, decision making, memory), energy disturbances (an increase with agitation/restlessness or a decrease with fatigue), feelings of excessive worthlessness or guilt, hopelessness, recurring thoughts about death or suicide or actual suicidal behavior.

Officially, according to the diagnostic manual of the American Psychiatric Association,* five or more of these signs or symptoms are required to make the formal diagnosis of a major depressive episode. It is important to note, however, that you do not need to have an "official," formal diagnosis of a major depressive episode in order to be treated. If you have some, not necessarily five or more, of these associated signs and symptoms (especially if they are interfering with your functioning or quality of life), you should be evaluated for treatment.

"Clinical depression" is a commonly heard term. It is a useful concept that refers, in general, to any depression that is severe enough to warrant treatment. It helps differentiate the *illness* depression from the normal "downs" and mild depressed moods that everybody experiences at times, that don't last long, that don't significantly interfere with functioning or quality of life, and that aren't accompanied by these other signs and symptoms.

There is an unofficial subtype of depression referred to as "masked depression." Masked depression is not listed in the official diagnostic manual, but all doctors know the term. People with this type of depression do not really feel down, blue, or melancholy. They often protest that they do not have depression because they do not *feel* depressed. However, they do have a number of the associated symptoms (described above) of the illness depression, and they frequently have physical symptoms also. Unexplained physical symptoms, for which the doctor can find no cause, are clues that lead a doctor to consider masked depression. People with masked depression frequently have pain, such as headaches or stomachaches or back pain, though the pain can actually be in any location. And though they doubt that they truly have depression, people with masked depression are often willing to at least give treatment a try when they are informed that treatment can give them relief.

The illness depression strikes people of all ages (children, adolescents, adults, and seniors), and females are two to three

---

* American Psychiatric Association, *Diagnostic and Statistical Manual of Mental Disorders,* Fourth Edition. (American Psychiatric Press, Washington, DC, 1994).

times more commonly affected than males. One out of every four women and one out of every ten men will suffer from the illness depression at some point in life. Yet it is horribly under-recognized, undiagnosed, and untreated, and about 15 percent of the people with untreated depression kill themselves rather than go on living in such misery.

Some of the official subtypes of depression are called major depressive disorder; dysthymic disorder; bipolar disorder, depressed phase; cyclothymic disorder; adjustment disorder with depressed mood; depression with psychotic features; depression with catatonic features; depression with melancholic features; depression with atypical features; depression with postpartum onset; and depression with seasonal pattern (commonly referred to as seasonal affective disorder syndrome, or SADS). Depression can also result from a medical condition (like Cushing's disease), a medication, or a "recreational" drug. Any and all of these subtypes may be treated with antidepressant medication. Delving into these subtypes, however, is beyond the scope of this book. For more information on the illness depression, please refer to the references in the Further Reading section at the end of the book.

3
_____

What Else Are the
Antidepressants Used For?

THE ANTIDEPRESSANTS, best known for treating depression,
are commonly used for treating other conditions as well.
What else are they used for, and how did these other uses come
about?

Once a medication enters our system, it goes all over our
body—not just to where we want it to go and no place else. At
times this results in an undesired effect on a bodily function.
When this happens, we think of it as a side effect (see Chapter
30, "What About Side Effects?"). At other times the medicine
has a simultaneous, positive effect on another different bodily
function. An example of this is a heart medicine that works not
only directly on the heart to help it pump more efficiently but
also on the blood pressure regulating system to help lower the
blood pressure. Sometimes medicines have positive effects in
totally unrelated areas of the body (or at least what *appear* to be
unrelated areas of the body). An example of this is aspirin: two
aspirins taken every four hours can help relieve a headache, and

one aspirin taken once daily can reduce blood clotting and the chances of a stroke or heart attack.

Since antidepressants have been around for over forty years, it is not surprising that other uses for them have been discovered. For treatment of "pure" anxiety, called generalized anxiety disorder, antianxiety medications have usually been the medicine of first choice, but some antidepressants have been shown to be just as effective. Historically, using an antidepressant in treating anxiety has generally been reserved for times when an antianxiety medicine can't be taken—in people with alcoholism, for example—or when the antianxiety medicine hasn't been effective. However, for years, antidepressants have been successful at treating anxiety mixed with depression, and in recent years, their success in treating panic attacks has been almost miraculous. In 1999, the antidepressant Effexor was approved by the FDA for treatment of generalized anxiety disorder. The antidepressants have also been useful as an adjunct in treating social phobia, eating disorders, and post-traumatic stress disorder, and Paxil has FDA approval for use in treating social phobia.

Furthermore, they have been used for years in other areas of medicine. Family practitioners, internists, and neurologists prescribe them regularly for the treatment of headaches and chronic pain. Pediatricians as well as child psychiatrists use them for treating conditions as different as bed-wetting and attention-deficit/hyperactivity disorder, which may also be treated by an antidepressant when it persists into adulthood.

Some of the new generation antidepressants, with their more precise effect on brain chemistry, are effective in relieving the symptoms of obsessive-compulsive disorder and obsessive-compulsive-related disorders (see below). Interestingly, they have also been shown to reduce the level of anger associated with some psychiatric disorders, and exciting research is pursuing this area. Furthermore, women who suffer from premenstrual dysphoric disorder (not just your "ordinary" premenstrual syndrome, but severe PMS with impairment in functioning) have found that some of these new generation antidepressants give them relief from their periodic suffering. Some men with premature ejaculation have also been treated successfully with them.

The U.S. Food and Drug Administration is very restrictive about what they allow a pharmaceutical company to claim on the drug's labeling and package insert. This is a good thing. It informs the citizenry about what illnesses or conditions that medicine has been shown, under strict scientific scrutiny, to effectively treat. However, the FDA recognizes that medicines are often useful in treating other conditions besides the one on the label. Therefore, it does not restrict doctors from using medicines for "other reasons." This is referred to as "off-label" prescribing, and doctors do it all the time. Some of the new generation antidepressants have even received "on-label" approval by the FDA for use in obsessive-compulsive disorder, panic disorder, generalized anxiety disorder, and bulimia nervosa.

The remainder of this chapter provides brief summaries of the other conditions treated by antidepressants. For more detailed information about them, see the list of references in the Further Reading section at the end of this book.

Obsessive-Compulsive Disorder

People with obsessive-compulsive disorder (OCD) are plagued by obsessions and/or compulsions. Obsessions are thoughts, ideas, impulses, or mental images that keep coming back and will not go away, even when the person tries to ignore, stifle, or resist them. Not always, but at some points in time, they cause significant distress or dysfunction, are recognized as unreasonable or excessive, and are experienced as intrusive and unwanted. They are different from worrying about real-life problems and are often senseless, unpleasant, distasteful, or even repugnant. Obsessions commonly involve one of the following issues: germs, contamination, or environmental toxins; someone getting sick, hurt, or killed; violence or aggression; sex; orderliness, symmetry, or exactness; religion or blasphemy; nonsense sounds, words, or numbers.

Compulsions are behaviors that the person feels driven (compelled) to do again and again, that are usually connected somehow to the person's obsessions, and that keep coming back and will not go away even when the person tries to ignore, stifle, or resist them. The intent of compulsions is often to prevent from happening whatever it is that the person is afraid of or obsessed about. The behavior itself, though, is way out of proportion to what is necessary, or it may be irrational in that it does not even make sense as to how it could accomplish what it is supposed to do. Examples of out-of-proportion behaviors include cleaning (e.g., hand washing, bathing, housecleaning) and "checking" (doors, locks, appliances). Examples of irrational compulsive behaviors include repeating a certain superstitious ritual, touching, collecting, arranging, hoarding, and saving. Often the behaviors must be done exactly according to certain "rules" the ill person has. And these behaviors do not necessarily have to be *physical* acts. They can be mental acts such as counting silently, repeating words in one's head, or silent prayer. As with obsessions, at some point they cause significant distress or dysfunction, are recognized as irrational or out of proportion, and are experienced as unwanted.

OCD is technically a subtype of the anxiety disorders, and anxiety is usually the emotional fuel that feeds the obsessive thoughts and compulsive behaviors. Behind almost every obsessive thought or compulsive behavior is a *fear* that something bad might happen.

Until recent years, OCD was thought to be a fairly rare condition. Now we know that it is not. The previous miscalculation was largely due to the sufferers' feelings of embarrassment about their unusual symptoms, which they kept secret from others. Nowadays, even when they know it is an illness and nothing to be ashamed of, patients are still reluctant to tell others about their symptoms. If you have OCD, do not feel alone: about 2 percent of the United States population (roughly

5 million people) have OCD. It usually hits people early in life (childhood, adolescence, or early adulthood).

OCD-Related Disorders

Also referred to as OCD-spectrum disorders, these illnesses are similar to OCD and may be treated by antidepressant medication. Eight subtypes are described below.

I. TRICHOTILLOMANIA

In everyday language, this disorder is referred to as compulsive hair pulling. People with trichotillomania are driven to pull out their hair, which they do to the extent that it is noticeable (not just a few plucks). As with other compulsions, the impulse keeps coming back, and the person suffering from it feels the tension to do it gradually build until it is unbearable. Attempts to ignore, stifle, or resist the impulse are unsuccessful. Relief is obtained only when the impulse is gratified by pulling out the hair. The site may be the head and/or other sites such as the eyebrows, arms, or pubic region.

Trichotillomania usually begins in childhood or adolescence. Like OCD, it is not as rare as we used to think, and may affect 1–2 percent of the population.

II. BODY DYSMORPHIC DISORDER

People with body dysmorphic disorder (BDD) believe they have, and are preoccupied with, what they think is some kind of defect in their personal appearance. The concern is so exaggerated and blown out of proportion that it causes them a great deal of discomfort. If there actually *is* something noticeably different about their appearance, their extreme preoccupation and exaggerated concern about it is what sets them apart from normal. People without BDD may be somewhat self-conscious about a bodily imperfection, but people with BDD are fanatic about it. Because of their extreme sensitivity about their "defect," social situations are quite difficult for them. The mere anticipation of social situations triggers anxiety, and they often find excuses not to participate. As you can imagine, this affects their daily functioning and keeps them from having what would otherwise be a normal life. A fair number of these people will go to a plastic surgeon hoping to get their "defect" corrected.

Body dysmorphic disorder has also been referred to as "imagined ugliness." Its extent in the general population is unknown.

III. HYPOCHONDRIASIS

People suffering with hypochondriasis automatically jump to the conclusion that they have a serious disease, regardless of how mild or insignificant their symptoms may be. Most of them make many trips to the doctor and undergo multiple physical examinations and medical tests. Despite repeated reassurances by the doctor that they have no major illness, the person's fears or thoughts persist. Often the medical workup finds absolutely nothing to explain their symptoms, but this lack of a specific medical diagnosis does not make a dent, and they remain preoccupied with their exaggerated illness.

IV. DEPERSONALIZATION DISORDER

Depersonalization (not necessarily depersonalization *disorder*) is the sensation of being detached from, or outside of, one's self. It is actually a fairly common experience, often described by such comments as "It seemed as if I was watching what was happening from someplace outside my body" and "It was like I was in a movie" (or a dream). Although it is experienced as a very strange feeling when it is happening, people remain in contact with reality and know that they are not *really* outside their body.

Depersonalization occurs often enough in the general population that it is not really considered pathological unless it causes the person significant distress or interferes with daily functioning. Depersonalization is a frequent occurrence during intense stress, during panic attacks, and in the course of other psychiatric illnesses. Depersonalization *disorder* itself (not just the *symptom* depersonalization) is diagnosed when the phenomenon of depersonalization occurs again and again in the absence of another psychiatric illness.

V. KLEPTOMANIA

People with kleptomania do not steal things for their personal use, for the benefit of friends, for resale, or for their monetary value. Often the objects are discarded or put away somewhere and never used. Neither are the objects stolen from a particular person in order to get revenge against that person. People with kleptomania are driven to steal things by an inner tension or an impulse that gathers strength until an object is stolen. As with trichotillomania, relief is obtained only when the impulse is gratified (in this disorder, by stealing the object). Kleptomania is all about the *act* of stealing, not about whatever is stolen.

VI. PATHOLOGICAL GAMBLING

Pathological gamblers are different from ordinary gamblers by virtue of their lack of control over their gambling. They are mentally obsessed with gambling, and their compulsive drive to gamble keeps returning, despite their efforts to ignore, stifle, or resist it. They often become restless or irritable when they try to cut back or quit. Eventually, in order to get enough excitement, they will increase their stake or the amount of time they spend gambling. Unable to quit and in an attempt to win back what they lost, they gamble even more. Sooner or later, they lie, obtain somebody else's money, or commit illegal acts so they can continue their gambling. If allowed to progress unchecked, the disorder will take over all other aspects of the afflicted person's life and leave it in ruins.

Pathological gambling affects men more often than women (a 2:1 ratio) and may be present in as much as 2 percent of the population of the United States.

VII. SEXUAL ADDICTIONS

Technically, there is no diagnosis of "sexual addiction" in the official psychiatric diagnostic manual. However, the term "sex addict" is commonly used, and the concept has received popular acceptance. People afflicted with sexual addictions are preoccupied with sex and are driven to gratify exaggerated or inappropriate sexual impulses. The antidepressants are sometimes used in treating these sexual disorders.

VIII. COMPULSIVE BUYING

As with the sexual addictions, there is no formal diagnosis of "compulsive buying" (also called compulsive shopping or compulsive spending) in the official psychiatric diagnostic manual. However, some sort of disorder in this area exists. It has yet to be adequately researched and understood. It is helpful to compare compulsive buying to kleptomania, except the impulse is to *buy* (not steal). The items bought are not needed and cost more than can actually be afforded, and uncontrollable indebtedness or bankruptcy frequently results.

Panic Disorder

People with panic disorder are plagued by repeated attacks of intense fear or panic. The attacks peak rapidly (within minutes) and involve some or most of the following symptoms: pounding heart, palpitations, or rapid heartbeat; sweating; shaking or trembling; shortness of breath or a feeling of choking or being smothered; chest discomfort or pain; abdominal distress or nausea; feeling dizzy, unsteady, light-headed, or faint; fear of losing control or going crazy; fear of dying; sensations of numbness or tingling; chills or hot flashes; feeling that things are not real; and feeling as if one is outside of one's self or detached (depersonalization). Technically, to make the formal diagnosis, at least four of these associated symptoms are necessary, and the attacks must have been coming and going for at least the past month. Some people have them for years before they seek professional help.

The panic attacks "come out of nowhere" and almost always leave the afflicted person afraid of, and worried about, having another one. When experiencing their first panic attack (and sometimes later panic attacks too), many people go to an emergency room, where they arrive hyperventilating and thinking they are having a heart attack. Once they learn about the disorder, such trips are not necessary.

Panic attacks may also be related to caffeine, to medical illnesses (e.g., hyperthyroidism), to medications (e.g., asthma medicine), or to alcohol and recreational drugs. Although such attacks may feel the same as the attacks of panic disorder, they are different and are not treated with the antidepressants.

Panic disorder may or may not be accompanied by agoraphobia, the fear of being in a place from which escape may be difficult or embarrassing, or in which help may not be available. Common places that agoraphobics fear include anywhere outside of home alone, or in a crowd, a shopping mall, restaurant, church, department store, an elevator, or on a bridge. Public transportation vehicles (buses, trains, planes), standing in a line, and being in a meeting or a classroom are other situations that agoraphobics fear and therefore avoid.

More women than men get panic disorder, and it can begin at any age (though onset in the elderly is rare). It affects 1–2 percent of the population.

Generalized Anxiety Disorder

People with generalized anxiety disorder (GAD) are plagued by ongoing, excessive anxiety and worry that is difficult to control. These excess anxieties and worries are not focused and limited to one thing (such as being contaminated, having another panic attack, being embarrassed in public), but are about a number of things (usually about routine aspects of life). Most everybody worries *a little* about these things, but for people with GAD, the anxieties and worries are distressful, interfere with daily functioning, and won't go away. They've been there for six months or longer (often for years), and though they may not be there every day, they're there more days than not. The focus of the anxiety and worry may shift from time to time, and the intensity may fluctuate, but the disorder itself is ongoing and often worsens in times of stress. The anxieties and worries are accompanied by associated symptoms such as disturbed sleep; feeling restless, keyed up, or on edge; irritability; difficulty in concentrating or the mind "going blank"; muscle tension; and susceptibility to fatigue.

GAD will affect 5 percent of Americans at some point in their life. It strikes women more often than men.

Social Phobia

People with social phobia are plagued by the fear of being in a situation in which they might do something that embarrasses or humiliates themselves in front of others. Common examples include the fear of speaking in public and being unable to finish the talk, fear of eating in a public place and choking on the food, fear of "freezing up" and being unable to urinate in a public rest room, fear of writing or signing one's name in public, fear of saying something foolish or being unable to answer questions.

Being in the feared situation will quickly trigger a panic attack, or at least a great deal of anxiety. Sufferers will therefore avoid such situations if they can. And if they can't avoid such a situation and must go through with it, they do so with intense internal distress.

Some symptoms of social phobia are not uncommon in the general population, though they are not severe enough to disrupt people's lives. However, at least 2 percent of Americans suffer from social phobia to the extent that it interferes with daily functioning and normal living. Social phobia often begins around puberty or adolescence, and women are more susceptible to it than men.

Eating Disorders

People with eating disorders place too much emphasis on their weight and body shape in determining their self-esteem and worth as a person and resort to desperate and unhealthful measures to keep from gaining weight. Those with bulimia intend to, and usually do, keep their weight on the low side (though not as low as anorexics). Those with anorexia nervosa are deeply afraid of getting fat and keep their weight so abnormally low that it is dangerous to their health. Amazingly, they do not see themselves as being that thin or emaciated and consequently don't realize the seriousness of their condition. Both bulimics and anorexics prevent weight gain by using such means as abnormal fasting and starvation, self-induced vomiting, excessive exercising, enemas, misuse of medications (laxatives, water pills, diet pills), and chewing their food but spitting it out before swallowing. Preoccupation with their appearance and weight consumes much of their mental energy. Many bulimics and anorexics will periodically go on binges, during which they feel they cannot control themselves and eat a huge amount of food. Additionally, anorexics will experience an absence of menstruation.

Surveys have shown that an eating disorder will affect at least 1–4 percent of all women at some point in their lives. Women are ten times more likely than men to have an eating disorder, which usually begins in adolescence or early adulthood.

Attention-Deficit/Hyperactivity Disorder

People with attention–deficit/hyperactivity disorder (ADHD) have had their symptoms since before grade school and, in some cases, since they were a baby. There are two main components of this illness: symptoms of inattention/distractibility and symptoms of hyperactivity/impulsivity. The inattention/distractibility component may be much stronger than the hyperactivity/impulsivity component, or vice versa, but usually there is a balanced mix. Symptoms of the inattention/ distractibility component include insufficient attention to detail when working on tasks, frequently resulting in careless mistakes; difficulty in sustaining attention and lack of follow-through, whether at work or play; avoidance of activities that require sustained attention (e.g., schoolwork); being easily distracted by other stimuli; difficulty in organizing things; forgetting things; appearing not to listen when spoken to; and losing things. Symptoms of the hyperactivity/impulsivity component include fidgeting or squirming; difficulty in remaining seated; frequently being "on the go"; restlessness; difficulty in playing quietly; excessive talking; interrupting others; and an impaired ability to wait one's turn.

Attention-deficit/hyperactivity disorder affects boys more often than it affects girls and has been estimated to occur in roughly 4 percent of school-age children. Contrary to what was believed ten or twenty years ago, many people with ADHD carry their disease with them into adulthood; not all kids outgrow ADHD during their teen years.

Post-Traumatic Stress Disorder

Post-traumatic stress disorder (PTSD) is a complex of signs and symptoms that arises in somebody who has been exposed to a horrifying event involving death, serious injury, or a threat of serious injury to self or others. People with PTSD never "got over what happened" and continue to have intense psychological or physical distress when reminded of the event, and/or distressing dreams or intrusive recollections of the event, and/or feelings that the event is recurring. People with PTSD have many of the following signs and symptoms: an exaggerated startle response; excessive vigilance; difficulty in concentrating; irritability; insomnia; decreased interest in activities; blunted emotions; feelings of detachment from others; a sense of a foreshortened future (i.e., the sufferer does not expect to have a normal life span); amnesia for part of the traumatic event; and avoidance of things (thoughts, feelings, activities, places, people, conversations) that are reminders of, or are associated with, the traumatic event.

This completes the brief descriptions of the psychiatric disorders that may be treated by the antidepressants. Let's move on and find out more about the antidepressants themselves.

4

Pills, Panaceas, and Placebos

A PANACEA IS A CURE-ALL. It is a mythical concept, because there is, in reality, no such thing. The Greeks coined the term centuries ago, but the concept has probably been around since the dawn of man. Witness Stone Age cultures and their medicine men performing rituals with various plants or animal parts. Witness the traveling huckster in America's Old West, selling bottles of "snake oil" and similar elixirs from the back of his medicine show wagon. It seems to be part of our human nature to hope that some type of medicine, or *something,* will cure all our ills.

The antidepressants are not panaceas. The antidepressants can relieve the symptoms of depression and the other illnesses mentioned in Chapter 3, but they won't make someone happy all the time.

Antidepressants can help bring someone up from depression into a normal mood. They can help reduce the ongoing suffering of those with obsessive-compulsive disorders. They can help diminish or even eliminate attacks of panic, symptoms of social phobia, and the frazzled nerves of the anxiety-ridden. They can help the abnormal thinking and behaviors of the eating disordered and reduce the distractibility/impulsivity of those with ADHD. They can help alleviate chronic pain and reduce the suffering of people with chronic headaches. They may help some women with severe PMS. But they cannot protect someone from having the occasional bad moods or bad days that everybody has, or the normal pains and sorrows that we all experience from time to time.

It is understandable to wish for a drug that can keep us free from emotional pain or psychological distress, but patients taking antidepressants must not set their hopes too high (as occasionally happens). There are no panaceas.

A placebo is an inactive medication, one that is inert and has no effects of its own. What is called the placebo effect is the result or impact that comes not from the actual chemical action of the medication, but from a person's psychological *expectation* of what that drug will do. How the placebo effect works is illustrated by how drunk fifteen-year-old Fred got the first time he drank.

✿ Case Example

Fred's parents were going for an overnight visit to Fred's uncle's in another town. They were normal, loving parents—maybe a little naive, but they'd had no experiences in the past that would lead them to mistrust Fred or suspect that Fred and his best friend weren't responsible and mature enough to stay home by themselves. However, they didn't know that Ann was having a slumber party that same night. Ann and Fred had attended grade school together and were now going to the same high school, and Fred had a crush on Ann. Fred's parents also did not know that some of the upperclassmen at Fred's high school had reputations as heavy weekend drinkers. These upperclassmen also happened to be athletic, good-looking, and popular with the girls (an observation that did not go unnoticed by Fred).

Fred thought he was pretty smart, and as his parents drove merrily on their way, he thought he was looking at the opportunity of a lifetime. His best friend couldn't have agreed more. A barely used bottle of vodka stood waiting in Fred's father's liquor cabinet. The boys poured a few ounces into an empty RC cola bottle, then poured a like amount of water back into the vodka bottle so that his father wouldn't notice the missing booze. Very clever they were. And they were going to be quite impressive to the girls at the slumber party.

After nightfall, they walked toward Ann's house, passing the cola bottle back and forth to each other and sipping the vodka whenever they reached the midway point between two streetlights. By the time they reached Ann's house, Fred was thinking he was pretty cool. He also thought he was drunk, though he had probably only swilled about two or three ounces of vodka. He swayed a little when Ann came to the door, then swaggered and staggered as the girls herded the two gentleman callers into the basement (away from Ann's parents).

A new Fred was born that night. Previously shy and reserved, Fred had the girls laughing until they cried. He danced with all of them. He danced by himself. He fell down. He teased them all and told jokes he didn't know he could remember, then laughed loudly—knowing he was the funniest person he knew. He knocked over a few chairs. He even announced in front of everybody, albeit with a thickened tongue, that he not only wanted *to take Ann out on a date, but he was* going to. *Several hours later he finally passed out—sprawled out on the floor except for his head, which was propped up in the corner of the room, chin placed perfectly in the middle of his chest.*

It is unlikely that just a few ounces of vodka accounted for all of Fred's drunken behavior. Surely his mind-set of what alcohol does to people in general, and his expectation of what alcohol would do to him, also influenced his antics. He was "under the influence" of more than just alcohol. He had also been influenced by the placebo effect.

Because we humans universally possess hopes, wishes, and fears of what a medicine will do to us, and because these expectations actually *do* influence what happens after we take a medicine, and also because some things happen just by coincidence after we take a medicine, all medications are scientifically investigated to find out which effects are just coincidence or placebo effects, and which effects are actually due to the medication. In fact, for every prescription drug in the United States that finally becomes available for usage today, an unbelievable amount of time and money is spent on research and development. It took an average of $359 million and 14.8 years for a new medicine to become available for prescription use in 1990.

One type of study performed on every new medicine is the "placebo-controlled study," in which a group of patients is given either the real medicine being investigated or an inactive placebo (usually sugar or a similar inert substitute). In a "blind" placebo-controlled study, the real medicine and the placebo are placed in identical-looking capsules, so patients don't know which one they are receiving.

One drawback of these blind placebo-controlled studies is that the doctor prescribing the medicine, or the nurse dispensing the medicine, knows what the patient is actually receiving. Unintentionally, the doctor or nurse may subtly give clues to patients about what they are taking, thus revealing the secret and ruining the scientific setup. In a "double-blind" placebo-controlled study, the identical-appearing capsules are coded and logged *before* they are given to the doctors and nurses so that neither the patients nor the doctors and nurses know which is the placebo and which is the real medicine. Once all the data from the study are in, the code is "broken" to see how the active medicine compared to the placebo. *All* possible effects are investigated: desired effects, undesired effects, side effects, chemical effects on the body and its organs, and so on.

All the antidepressants have been thoroughly researched, including rigorous, double-blind placebo-controlled studies. This is great news for patients who are frightened or skeptical of taking an antidepressant. No drug ever comes close to being released on the market without having clear, documented proof of its effectiveness and safety.

Another advantage of this research is the huge databank that accumulates and is recorded about each drug. Important statistics are available on every antidepressant, so that patients do not have to (and *should not*) draw too many conclusions from what happened to the one or two people they know who took the drug. Too often people think that because Aunt Tillie or their friend Billy developed such and such effects after taking a medicine, they, too, are likely to develop such and such if they take that medicine. The statistics based on double-blind placebo-controlled studies of hundreds or thousands of patients will dispel rumor and give you an accurate idea of what to expect.

5

The Pendulum: Psychological
and Chemical Imbalances

NOT TOO LONG AGO, many people preferred psychotherapy over psychiatric medication. They wanted to "get at the underlying psychological problem." They didn't want to subject their brain to drugs that hadn't yet received public acceptance. The legacy of Sigmund Freud and psychoanalysis led many to hope that, by delving deeply into their unconscious mind, they could lead a happier life and achieve better health. The success and effectiveness of the various psychotherapeutic methods spread by word of mouth. People with psychiatric disorders came in with their mind made up about treatment: they wanted psychotherapy and they did not want medication.

Furthermore, some people (although they were already in relatively good mental health) sought professional help to "get even better." All types of mental health professionals, no matter what particular training they had received, contributed to this trend by gladly supplying their particular brand of psychotherapy, with good intentions, to those who wanted it.

Nowadays, the pendulum has swung the other way. Many

people prefer medication over psychotherapy. Who has not heard of Prozac and the wonderful things it has done? Isn't it only human to harbor some wishful thinking that merely taking a medicine once a day will lead to a happier life and better mental health? Wouldn't it be nice to just pop a pill and not have to face the unpleasant realities that will inevitably occur in life? Consider the following anecdote.

✿ Case Example

Ellie, a fairly bright woman, came into the psychiatrist's office requesting an antidepressant for her depression. Ellie made it clear that she did not want any counseling or psychotherapy. She wanted to "just try an antidepressant for a month or two and see what happens." Two of her friends, and a few more of her friends' friends, previously had depression and improved while on antidepressants. Ellie had read magazine articles and books about depression and had seen the warning signs listed on TV. Indeed, she had quite a few of the warning signs and told her doctor about them. She felt unhappy much of the time and was tense and irritable. Her appetite had diminished, and she frequently felt as if she had a knot in her stomach (plus, she had lost some weight). She had some trouble falling asleep at night and felt tired during the day. Her desire to have sex with her husband was zero. She had difficulty in concentrating; instead, she was preoccupied with her situation. There was a positive family history too: her mother's sister had many signs of depression for years (though she had never been treated). Ellie said the problems in her life were "no more than the usual" and described her relationship with her husband as "normal, about like the average marriage."

However, a more detailed, hour-long history from Ellie was revealing. When asked more about her lack of sexual desire, a different picture began to emerge. It turned out that she had retained a healthy libido, but her sex drive for her husband was nonexistent. Somewhat offhandedly, she commented, "Actually, I think I'd rather punch his lights out than make love with him."

This statement gave her doctor an opening to further explore

Ellie's marriage. Just minutes before, she had maintained that her marriage was okay, and had shifted the conversation to something else. Now she began to open up some about her husband. Ellie's husband was a meticulous and conscientious engineer. He had high standards and he stuck to them. He was loyal and dedicated to his family (including Ellie) and his employer, and he was known throughout the community as a good man. He would work fifty or sixty hours a week when it was necessary to "do the job right," which was pretty much the rule. He also spent a fair amount of time working around the yard and the house, and he was a dependable volunteer at their church. Ellie appreciated her husband. He was a good provider, and his character was without a blemish. He was not the most romantic of men, however, and she admitted that, in fact, he was frequently distant and cold. His thoughts seemed to be somewhere else, and he always had "something more to do."

Ellie went on. It seemed her husband had some very firm beliefs about what a wife's duties are. Over the years, Ellie had tried to change how they "divided up the labor" around the house, but her husband wouldn't hear of it. Arguing that he "worked his tail off and never complained," he couldn't see how she could complain about "just a few responsibilities around the house." After six years of marriage, they were in a stalemate. Ellie was crying now as she continued. Over the last two years, every time Ellie brought the subject up, or even mildly complained about something in the course of her doing her "duties," her husband would become infuriated. So Ellie fulfilled her responsibilities around the home and didn't complain. Peace was kept and they didn't fight. She did her thing and he did his, and they got along. "Sure," Ellie admitted, "it could be better, but no marriage is perfect." She began regaining her composure. "Our marriage is as good as the next guy's, and I really don't think that's the problem. Nor do I think anything can be done about it. I think I'm just depressed, and I would like to try an antidepressant."

How much was Ellie's depression caused by her marital problems and suppressed feelings? How much was she, in her depressed state, being supersensitive or exaggerating the situation? We will never know; she never returned. We do know that Ellie (and her husband) could have benefited from more than just an antidepressant. It doesn't take a psychiatrist to figure that out.

Occasionally, patients or family members ask if there is some type of laboratory test that can tell whether or not a "chemical imbalance" exists in the brain. The availability of such a test would be magnificent. However, there is no test that can be performed on a patient's blood, urine, or cerebrospinal fluid in order to determine, with certainty, that a chemical imbalance in the brain does or does not exist. A laboratory procedure called the dexamethasone suppression test (DST) was, and still is, sometimes used to give doctors a clue about what is happening chemically in the brain. But it is nowhere near as meaningful as, say, a blood sugar test in diagnosing and treating diabetes. Furthermore, the outcome of the DST can be influenced by a variety of other factors. Scientists are aggressively researching tests, including the DST, that provide data about brain chemistry, but since a consistently reliable test has yet to be developed, diagnostic and treatment decisions are better if they are based on nonlaboratory information.

There are lab tests, though, that are used to help diagnose other medical illnesses that cause symptoms of depression, anxiety, and panic (see Chapter 11, "Medical Factors"). For example, blood tests can help detect illnesses such as thyroid disease and myasthenia gravis. Such tests may be recommended by your doctor so that the two of you are not fooled by another condition that mimics depression or anxiety. But they are not to be confused with the tests that will someday help us diagnose and monitor the chemical imbalances in the brain that occur with psychiatric illnesses.

Like Ellie, many people have hopes that a chemical imbalance is the sole problem and, therefore, a medication *by itself* will be the answer. Unfortunately, many doctors are actually contributing to this swing of the pendulum by gladly supplying (with good intentions) these wonderful drugs, but not delving any further into what's happening in their patients' life.

The vast majority of people who are taking antidepressant medications would do better if they *combined* their medication with appropriate psychotherapy. It does not have to be one or the other. In fact, research confirms that moderately and severely depressed people have a better outcome when treated with *both* medication and psychotherapy.

This is like "covering all the bases." Psychiatric treatment, like life, is not cut-and-dried, black or white. Combating psychiatric disorders is more likely to be successful by combining medication *and* psychotherapy.

6

"Mild" and "Strong" Antidepressants, and Milligrams

OCCASIONALLY, PATIENTS ASK if they could just try a "mild" antidepressant. They ask this when they are not in a great deal of emotional pain, when they are reluctant in general to take a medication, and when they are afraid to put anything "powerful" or unknown into their body. On the other hand, some patients do just the opposite and ask for a "strong" medicine. Sometimes they say, "Give me the strongest thing you've got."

There is no such thing as a "mild" or a "strong" antidepressant. No one antidepressant is any weaker than another, and no one is any stronger than another. No one works better for the "milder" cases, and no one works better for the "severe" cases.

Similarly, patients occasionally get overly concerned about the number of milligrams of the medication they are taking. They will see or hear that they are on a certain number of milligrams, then become unnecessarily anxious that they might be on too much or not enough medication.

🌿 Case Example

Richard's first panic attack occurred when he was around twenty. He distinctly remembers where he was driving on the beltway when it hit him. At first it was a combination of the shortness of breath and the fear. He thinks he remembers the shortness of breath coming first, but he is not sure. He knows the fear was there almost immediately: the fear that he couldn't get enough air and the feeling that he was suffocating. Panic hit. "Am I going to die? Am I having a heart attack? What is wrong with me?" He ended up going to an emergency room, where he was told he had hyperventilation and that nothing was really wrong with him or his heart.

In subsequent years, Richard had additional episodes consisting of shortness of breath, chest pain, sweating, and nervousness. He had been to several doctors, and his examinations, EKGs, and stress tests were always normal. One emergency room doctor told him that he had panic disorder and gave him a tranquilizer, which relieved his symptoms within an hour. Richard then found a family physician who prescribed him tranquilizers on an as-needed basis over the next several years.

In the last year, however, Richard's attacks had increased to where he was having them daily. His job had become more stressful due to a new boss who didn't like him and a dramatically increased workload. Richard's new wife felt rejected when he began spending more time at work, and she became sick and tired of hearing about his bodily complaints all the time. Not only was Richard having chest pain, he also complained of numbness and tingling, light-headedness, feeling "off-kilter," and a knot in his stomach. Richard returned to his family physician. When again his tests were normal, he was again told he had panic disorder. The tranquilizers gave him some relief, but the attacks would inevitably return. One day his family physician told him he was using too many tranquilizers and something more needed to be done. Richard was then referred to a psychologist.

The sessions with the psychologist proved helpful, but when

Richard still continued to have the attacks, the psychologist and the family doctor referred him to a psychiatrist for further consultation regarding his medication.

The psychiatrist added an antidepressant to Richard's medication regimen. The next morning, the psychiatrist received a telephone call from Richard's wife, who politely said she would like to ask the psychiatrist a few questions. "First," she asked, "why is Richard being treated with an antidepressant *when he clearly is having* anxiety *and not depression?" The psychiatrist explained to her how medications in general can have more than one use, and cited the example of how the anti-inflammatory drugs, which are primarily used for arthritic conditions, are also used for menstrual cramps. The psychiatrist went on to explain how antidepressant medication had been successfully used in treating panic attacks for more than fifteen years. Richard's wife grunted a "humpff, well . . ." and went on a long diatribe about what she had been through for the past year. Then she asked, clearly no longer able to conceal her skepticism, why Richard had been prescribed only 10 milligrams of the antidepressant. Her mother had been on 200 milligrams of an antidepressant, she said. "How is Richard ever going to get better on such a small number of milligrams? Isn't that like treating a bad headache with baby aspirin?"*

This patient's wife's misunderstanding was, as is usually the case, based on the assumption that the strength or potency of every milligram is the same for all drugs (i.e., 100 mg of one drug is equivalent to 100 mg of any other drug). Following this logic, one would conclude that 100 mg of one drug is ten times stronger than 10 mg of another drug, which is ten times stronger than 1 mg of a third drug. This logic is misleading. Before any drug comes on the market, researchers scientifically determine what is the probable number of milligrams that the average person will need in order to get the desired effect from that drug. This varies extremely from one drug to another, depending on the particular characteristics of each individual drug. The recommended starting dose may end up being a high, intermediate, or low number of milligrams. For example, a 150 mg dose per day may be perfect for one antidepressant (e.g., Tofranil) but may be subtherapeutic for another drug (e.g., Wellbutrin) or may even be an overdose of a third antidepressant (e.g., Nardil).

Using drugs in other areas of medicine can further illustrate the point of how different doses are effective regardless of the number of milligrams used: a typical dose of the heart medicine digitalis is 0.1 mg, and a typical dose of aspirin is 650 mg.

Each individual's unique physiology, genetic makeup, and brain chemistry also determine what is the proper dose for that individual (as you will see in Chapter 21, "Finding the Right Dose"). For example, two people could have identical symptoms of depression, of obsessive-compulsive disorder, or whatever, and the symptoms could be of equal severity. They could be treated with the same medication but, due to unique differences in their body chemistry, require an eightfold difference in the dosage needed to achieve symptom relief (e.g., one needing only 25 mg of Zoloft, the other needing 200 mg of Zoloft). Do not get worried about the number of milligrams of the medicine you are taking. Every medicine is different and every person is different.

7

Are the Antidepressants
Addicting?

PATIENTS AND THEIR FAMILY MEMBERS often ask if the antidepressants are addicting. No, they are not.

Addicting drugs cause "tolerance," whereby the brain needs more and more of the drug to get the same effect. Consider the example of the eighteen-year-old who gets a buzz from one or two beers when he first begins drinking alcoholic beverages. Three years and many, many beers later, it takes six beers for him to get the same buzz. That is tolerance.

The antidepressants do not cause tolerance. Once the effective dose is reached, your brain does not need a larger and larger daily dose in order to keep the desired effect. Occasionally, however, people who have been on a stable, continuous dose of an antidepressant do need their dose adjusted (usually upward). This is the depression "breaking through" the medicine, and such an event is the exception, not the rule. When it occurs, the dose or the medicine itself is changed in order to treat the breakthrough. It is important to know that this is not tolerance.

You will not need to keep taking higher and higher doses to keep your symptoms at bay.

Addicting drugs, when abruptly withheld, can leave the user with physical withdrawal symptoms. As a rule, this does not happen with the antidepressants. However, on some occasions, susceptible people will suffer "withdrawal" symptoms if the level of antidepressant in their blood drops too rapidly. This can happen when a few doses in a row are skipped, whatever the reason. When it does happen, it can make people feel sick, as if they have the flu. It is not dangerous or life-threatening, and fortunately, only a minority of the population is susceptible to this. Chapter 26, "How to Stop an Antidepressant" describes how you can avoid this happening to you.

Patients and family members should know that one's psychiatric symptoms may return after an antidepressant is discontinued. This may happen days, weeks, months, or years later. When and if this happens, it is not "withdrawal" from the medication, akin to "withdrawal" from heroin in a heroin addict. It is a return of the original illness, akin to an asthmatic individual having his asthma flare up after discontinuing his asthma medication.

Some susceptible individuals may need to take their medications for years, or even indefinitely. This will prevent a return of the symptoms and is called maintenance medication (see Chapter 25, "When and If to Stop an Antidepressant," and Chapter 36, "Relapses and Recurrences"). The good news about this is that the antidepressants can prevent people from having to go through recurrences, which is what they would do if these medicines were not available.

Technically, people on maintenance medication are dependent on their medicine. But taking long-term medication prescribed for an illness is not the same as an addict taking a drug long-term on his own (not as prescribed) in order to get high. You do not think of someone who is taking asthma medication as being "addicted," nor do you when the illness is diabetes, high blood pressure, or a disease of the heart or thyroid gland.

Taking maintenance medication for depression is no different from taking maintenance medication for these illnesses.

AN ARTIFICIAL HIGH?

Some patients say that they don't want to take an antidepressant medication because they don't want to be on an "artificial high" or an "unnatural high." Antidepressant medications do not cause an artificial high. They help bring someone who is down back up to normal. They help relieve the symptoms of depression, or the symptoms of the other illnesses mentioned in Chapter 3, but they do not push people into an *unnaturally* good mood.

The antidepressants are different from alcohol and recreational drugs. The antidepressants work on those key areas in the brain where the chemicals are essentially out of balance. Since their mechanism of action is dramatically different from that of alcohol and recreational drugs, there is no "buzz." Nobody parties with the antidepressant drugs. You never see a drug abuser using the antidepressant drugs to get high, and you never see these medications sold on the street. That ought to tell you something right there.

8

The Antidepressants
and Violence

PATIENTS OR FAMILY MEMBERS sometimes ask if the antidepressants cause violence or suicidal behavior. Plain and simple, no, they do not. There are many important things to talk about with your doctor, and there is so little time. Unless you really believe there might be some truth to this myth, don't waste your time and your doctor's time by asking questions about this. Regardless of what you may have heard or read about the antidepressants causing violence or suicide, the scientific facts show that there is absolutely no causation.

Most of the attention focused on this violence issue had to do with just one of the antidepressants (Prozac). And most of this stemmed from word-of-mouth rumor, lawsuits, a few tragedies that occurred when people happened to be taking Prozac, and one journal article. The subsequent media attention kept Prozac in the public's eye, and some people have been wary of Prozac ever since. To make matters worse, the Church of Scientology promoted a campaign and hyped this rumor in an effort to discredit Prozac. (Scientologists are followers of the late

L. Ron Hubbard and his belief system. They actively oppose psychiatrists and encourage people not to use psychiatric medicine, but to use the methods of their Scientology belief system instead.)

None of the accusations about Prozac causing violence or suicide has been proved to have any scientific merit, and none of the lawsuits has been successful. In fact, an FDA advisory committee (a panel of impartial experts) unanimously agreed that "there is no credible evidence of a causal link between the use of antidepressant drugs, including Prozac, and suicidality or violent behavior." Committee chairman Daniel E. Casey, M.D., also stated, "And regarding Prozac, we have looked more closely and analytically at those data than on any other antidepressant drug."*

In reality, suicidal thinking and behaviors *decrease* when patients are treated with Prozac, which is what happens with the other antidepressants as well.

A word of warning, however, is in order. Neither Prozac nor any antidepressant will work for everybody. People can and do get worse if the particular antidepressant they are taking is not working. Thoughts and impulses of suicide or violence can happen, and they can get worse if the antidepressant is not working. If and when such thoughts or impulses occur or increase, they should be reported to your doctor.

* Food and Drug Administration, Talk Paper (U.S. Department of Health and Human Services, 5600 Fishers Land, Rockville, MD, October 18, 1991).

What to Say to
the Doctor

9

The Therapeutic Alliance, Part I: Starting Out

B EFORE STARTING ANY ANTIDEPRESSANT, the patient should be completely open and honest with the physician. Together they form an alliance against the illness they are fighting. The odds of success depend highly on their teamwork and cohesiveness. No case of depression, OCD, panic disorder, or whatever is exactly like another. Everybody is different, and to treat all cases the same, boilerplate fashion, is not the best approach. The doctor should ask about, and the patient should tell about, the pertinent particulars of that patient's individual case. The doctor needs this information, for it is the data on which that patient's unique treatment plan will be based. The doctor must listen to the patient and hear what is said, before and during the course of treatment. If a doctor minimizes or discounts some of what a patient says, and then proceeds with a treatment plan that was previously set in the doctor's mind, then that particular treatment plan will not be individually tailored to that specific patient.

Similarly, if the patient does not provide all the proper information, then the physician cannot really obtain a comprehensive, thorough evaluation and is therefore forced to make a pharmacological decision with one hand tied behind his back. One of the essential things to know about being on any of these medications is that it may not work at all if the prescribing physician does not know about the particular characteristics of your case. Chapters 10 to 17 cover information you should discuss with your physician.

10

Signs and Symptoms

INEVITABLY, YOU WILL TELL your physician why you are there seeking help. You will tell him or her about your symptoms, about your "pain." This is good. The doctor needs to know all about your pain and all the sources of your pain. As patients describe their pain, they usually include painful events and painful relationships that have happened or are happening in their life. It is important for the doctor to know about these things. However, in doing an initial medication evaluation, the doctor does not need to hear all the nitty-gritty details of these events and relationships. These details may well be of vital importance, but they can be addressed later. The time allocated for the initial medication evaluation is better spent on gathering other information, including an "inventory" of current symptoms. From a pharmacological standpoint, it does not matter what the particular problems are that are causing the symptoms. The medication will work on your brain chemicals regardless of what painful events and relationships may have happened in your life. Your doctor needs to know your specific signs and symptoms.

Sometimes patients believe that certain events have caused their symptoms when, in fact, those events have not. By shifting the focus away from the theoretical or alleged causes (whether or not they really are the actual causes—see Chapter 33, "Cause and Effect") and focusing instead on the specific signs and symptoms from which you need relief, you can clarify for both the doctor and yourself what you are trying to change. It is helpful to identify "target symptoms." In what ways are your thoughts, feelings, emotions, bodily functions, and actions different from how you would like them to be? Such a symptom-focused approach can avoid the treatment error of erroneously pursuing what was thought to be the cause of the patient's symptoms (i.e., barking up the wrong tree).

Identifying and clarifying the target symptoms also helps to establish the proper diagnosis. If too much time and energy are spent discussing the situation thought to be *causing* the symptoms, and not enough time and energy are spent on accurately *diagnosing* the symptoms, treatment may not work. For example, consider the following.

🌿 CASE EXAMPLE

Danielle sought counseling for problems she was having with her husband. She had become increasingly unhappy over the past six months, and what used to be a minor stressor would now trigger a temper outburst and/or tears. She frequently found fault with, and complained to, her husband. Her husband became increasingly frustrated and told her it seemed to him as if he couldn't do anything right—she would always find something he did to get mad about. After the first few months of this, they agreed to try not to fight. They had been married almost twenty years, and both of them knew they loved each other. They sincerely tried to avoid fighting with each other, but the pattern repeated itself, and they had some "humdingers." Danielle found herself thinking about divorce. She was miserable. She realized that their efforts weren't working, and she decided to get some "outside help." A good friend of Danielle's referred her to Ms. Stanton, a therapist who had been a marvelous help to the friend a few years back.

In their second session, Ms. Stanton used the word "codependency," explained some of this concept to Danielle, and recommended that Danielle read a book about codependency. Danielle read the book and some of it seemed to apply to her. Over the next few months, Danielle and Ms. Stanton met weekly. Danielle learned more about codependency and worked hard to catch herself when she fell back into her old codependent habits. She did the homework assignments that Ms. Stanton gave her to do between sessions, made a conscious effort to view her relationship with her husband (and her entire world) from a new angle, and tried different approaches to problem solving and conflict resolution with her husband. Her husband came to a few sessions with her, also read the book, and was supportive of Danielle's efforts to not be so codependent. Unfortunately, though, Danielle remained unhappy. She was crying even more. At times, she began thinking she was a failure—at therapy and as a wife. Nothing pleased her, and she vacillated between blaming and getting angry at her husband and blaming and getting mad at herself.

As therapy progressed, Danielle and Ms. Stanton focused more on the issue of Danielle's self-esteem. The fact emerged that Danielle had not been 100 percent confident in herself for years, if ever. They traced her feelings of insecurity back to Danielle's childhood, when the insecurity began. They got into Danielle's relationship with her parents and the fact that Danielle's mother was a woman who was also difficult to please. There was plenty of "grist for the mill" in therapy, and Ms. Stanton proved to be a sensitive listener, an empathic and caring person, and a counselor who provided good, solid, down-to-earth advice, which Danielle really appreciated. Danielle did not want to just analyze and intellectualize on and on about the past (a process she termed "psychobabble"). Neither was she into Rolfing, primal screaming, or other therapeutic techniques that she considered far-out and gimmicky. Ms. Stanton was practical, and her counsel made good common sense; Danielle liked that.

Still, Danielle was unhappy. She and Ms. Stanton discussed

everything they could think of that could have been causing her emotional turmoil. During one session, Danielle confided to Ms. Stanton that she had been having thoughts about "just ending it all"; nothing seemed to be getting better. Ms. Stanton immediately referred Danielle to a psychiatrist for a second opinion and an evaluation for possible medication.

During the consultation with the psychiatrist, Danielle began telling the psychiatrist about the things her husband did that made her unhappy. As tactfully and gracefully as she could, the psychiatrist tried to direct Danielle away from these complaints about her husband and focus instead on what symptoms Danielle was having. Danielle described how miserable she was and began explaining how her self-esteem was down, that she had always had a little insecurity, and how it all related to her codependency, her childhood, her mother, etc. Patiently, the psychiatrist explained that she did not need to hear all that today. What she needed to hear today was more about Danielle's signs and symptoms.

That's when it came out that Danielle was sad and unhappy almost all the time. It seemed that she was unable to enjoy or experience pleasure from anything. It had been weeks since she had laughed. She had difficulty with concentrating during the day and difficulty in sleeping at night because her thoughts kept coming back to her deteriorating marriage, what a jerk her husband was, and what a jerk she had been for being so codependent. The psychiatrist politely shifted the focus from what Danielle had been thinking and crying about, both day and night, to the crying, the sleeplessness, the trouble with concentration, the irritability, and the suicidal thoughts as signs and symptoms of depression. She recommended an antidepressant to Danielle, and that Danielle continue her psychotherapy with Ms. Stanton.

Once the diagnosis of depression was made, and Danielle was treated with an antidepressant along with her psychotherapy, she dramatically improved.

Don't spend a disproportionate amount of your initial visit with the doctor talking about what you think is causing your signs and symptoms. Tell your doctor about your signs and symptoms themselves.

Sometimes the patient's signs and symptoms are glossed over during the initial medical evaluation because the patient has "already made the diagnosis." It is tempting, especially in the more medically informed society of today, to diagnose oneself, then say to the doctor, "I'm depressed; please treat me." The problem with this is that most people have not gone to medical school and have therefore not learned how to be properly vigilant and do not know what to look for in case something else is going on. And even if someone has had the proper training, one should not diagnose oneself because one cannot be objective about oneself. Everybody has blind spots.

🌿 Case Example

Dr. Joe was a busy doctor who had built a successful practice over the past twenty-five years and was loved by all of his patients. But things were changing. Some of his old patients were switching to other doctors—not because they were unhappy with Dr. Joe, but because of new insurance agreements their employers had entered into and the significant out-of-pocket dollars they would save by switching physicians. New patients quickly filled the appointments, so Dr. Joe wasn't hurt financially by these changes, but he did not like what was happening. Many of his old patients apologized for switching; some cried. Dr. Joe had joined some of the new insurance plans and managed-care agreements, but he didn't like them either. Gobs of paperwork and phone calls were required for "authorization" and "documentation." He felt harried during the day, realized he was hurrying his patients and their families out the door, and was still getting home later at night.

Things weren't the same at home anymore either. His children were all out of the nest now. The "baby" (his youngest daughter), a zippy and enthusiastic ball of energy who was crazy about her daddy, had left for college earlier this year.

Dr. Joe was tired. He was tired when he got up in the morning, he was tired at work, and he was tired when he got home in the evening. He used to love life and enjoy it to the fullest—now his zest was gone. It seemed that all he wanted to do was sleep, and he did sleep a lot more than usual. He was burned-out. He felt mentally dulled, and when the thought entered his head that he would just as soon be dead, he realized he had the symptoms of depression. He was constipated, and his libido was down as well. His wife agreed that he had seemed more withdrawn and depressed to her. Dr. Joe knew he couldn't single-handedly stop the changes in the health-care industry that were sweeping the country and affecting his practice. He also knew that it was best that his children move on with their own lives; it wouldn't be right to bring them back home just to treat his depression. What he could do, though, was take an antidepressant. He had plenty of samples at the office, and he began himself on the appropriate starting dose.

Several weeks later, however, Dr. Joe was no better. In fact, he felt more exhausted. Dr. Joe knew he probably shouldn't be treating himself, and he thought about calling a psychiatrist friend whom he respected and trusted, but the psychiatrist was awfully busy and Dr. Joe didn't want to be a bother. Besides, Dr. Joe had treated hundreds of patients for depression and he knew what to do next—up the dose. So he did.

A month later Dr. Joe had increased the dose once more and still felt depressed. His energy had dropped even more, and now he didn't know if it was the depression or the antidepressant that was making him more tired. Finally, he decided to do what he knew he should have done at the start—go to a doctor.

It was a good thing he did, because otherwise he may have gone on for months diagnosing and treating himself for depression when his primary problem was actually with his thyroid gland. Once his hypothyroidism was properly treated by an internist, Dr. Joe's symptoms resolved.

Doctors are, of course, human too and subject to the same foibles we all have. Whether you are a doctor or not, don't attempt to diagnose yourself. Let your doctor do that. Your job is to tell your doctor your signs and symptoms.

Besides identifying the specific target symptoms from which you want relief, it also helps to prioritize them. Frequently, patients talk on and on about the many symptoms they are having, going into endless detail about each symptom and how it is affecting their life. They are overwhelmed and it is easy to understand why. But a long speech about all the details of your symptoms can overwhelm your doctor, who is then left not knowing what bothers you the most. If you can prioritize your symptoms and tell your doctor which of your symptoms are the main ones you would choose to get relief from first, then those are what your doctor will focus on first.

11

Medical Factors

D R. JOE'S HYPOTHYROIDISM is but one example of how a medical condition can mimic depression. Many other medical conditions can cause symptoms of depression, panic, anxiety, and obsessive-compulsive disorder. Hyperthyroid and parathyroid conditions, Cushing's disease, lupus, strokes, Alzheimer's and other forms of dementia are additional examples. Infections such as Lyme disease can masquerade as depression. Mononucleosis, diabetes, hypoglycemia, anemia, AIDS, Parkinson's, and various types of cancer and tumors can also cause psychiatric symptoms. So can certain forms of epilepsy, electrolyte imbalances, and relatively uncommon illnesses such as Huntington's and Addison's. Any of these could go undiagnosed and therefore untreated. It is essential that, in such cases, these illnesses be undisguised and treated for what they really are.

   It is important to tell your physician about all medical conditions you currently have and about all your current symptoms—physical symptoms included. You should also tell your physician about medical conditions you have had in the past, because an illness you had previously may be flaring up again without you knowing it.

Medical conditions are not only important to know about when making a diagnosis, they are also a factor when it comes to choosing which antidepressant to use and how much of it to use. A disease affecting a major organ, such as the heart, kidney, or liver, should obviously be taken into consideration. Even a relatively minor condition, such as a blood pressure that tends to run a little low, may become a significant condition when taking an antidepressant.

The eating disorders (anorexia nervosa and bulimia nervosa) deserve special mention here. Not uncommonly, the patient's body chemistry (electrolyte balance in particular) is thrown off-base during the course of an eating disorder. When intentional vomiting or fasting is occurring, and especially when laxatives or diuretics are being abused, the patient *must* come clean and tell the doctor. Otherwise, a potentially dangerous interaction could occur between the medication and the altered body chemistry.

Don't try to weed out health information that you think is not relevant or that you don't want your doctor to know. Make sure your physician knows your entire medical history and let him or her be the judge of whether or not something is relevant.

12

Medications

B E SURE YOUR DOCTOR knows about all the medicines you
are currently taking, since sometimes medications cause
symptoms that mimic depression, panic, and anxiety. It is similar to how a medical illness sometimes masquerades as a psychiatric illness, as was described in the previous chapter. The
following case exemplifies why this can be important.

⚘ CASE EXAMPLE

*Mike came into the emergency room at 3:00 A.M. hyperventilat-
ing and complaining of light-headedness. He hadn't slept at all that
night, and his heart had been racing for two hours. He had been
getting more and more short of breath, but it was different from an
asthma-type shortness of breath, which Mike had experienced before.
Mike was scared; he wondered if something was wrong with his
heart. He was so nervous and restless that he was unable to sit still
for more than a minute without getting up and walking around. He*

was shaky, inside and out. His fingers and lips were tingling and partially numb.

A quick listen to Mike's chest confirmed that it was not asthma, and the emergency room physician reassured Mike that the preliminary diagnosis was a panic attack and not anything serious. "But I'm going to check you out thoroughly and make sure it is not your heart or something else," she told Mike. Mike checked out okay, but the thorough and astute emergency room physician picked up on something Mike said, and began asking him more questions. Mike's asthma and allergies had, in fact, been bothering him in the past two weeks. He had gone to a neighborhood medical clinic and had received a prescription for some steroid medication. Additionally, Mike had been using an old inhaler from his medicine cabinet and some over-the-counter decongestants he bought at the drugstore. Mike had no idea exactly how much of these medicines he had used over the past few days, but he reassured the doctor that he had not taken more than what the instructions said to take.

After a tranquilizer, reassurance from the physician that nothing serious was wrong, and a few hours, Mike's symptoms began to subside. Before he went home, Mike was again reassured that he'd had a panic attack and that he was physically fine. However, no referral to a psychiatrist was made and no prescriptions were written. "Mike, I think your panic attack was medication-induced. I recommend you consult with a doctor and get your asthma under good medical control, then see if you have any more panic attacks." Mike did this and had no further panic attacks. He never needed an antidepressant, a tranquilizer, or any psychiatric treatment.

The medicines most notorious for having side effects of anxiety and depression are high blood pressure medicines, asthma medicines, and steroids (i.e., prednisone and other medicines related to cortisone). Many other medicines can also do it, but we will not publish a list of such medicines and have you try to diagnose yourself. Besides, with new medications coming out on the market every week, such a list would be quickly outdated. It is best just to make sure your physician knows about every medicine you are taking, even if it is only occasionally, and even if it is an over-the-counter, nonprescription drug.

13

Previous Treatment

I F A PATIENT had a positive response to one particular antidepressant in the past, and the illness is flaring up again, it is likely the physician will prescribe that same medication again, especially if there were no significant side effect problems the first time. Stick with a winner.

CASE EXAMPLE

Linda came to a psychiatrist for help with depression. She was informed and knowledgeable about the psychiatric disorders and had "diagnosed" herself several weeks earlier when she realized she felt like crying almost daily and didn't feel like doing anything anymore. She also recognized the associated symptoms of fatigue and trouble with sleeping. She initially thought the fatigue was due to her not sleeping well, so she tried some melatonin and later some over-the-counter sleeping medicines. Sometimes they helped, but she was still tired the next day, even when she'd had a decent night's sleep the night before.

The psychiatrist took a thorough history and performed a partial physical examination. Linda was in good health and had no past or current illnesses that the psychiatrist could identify as possibly contributing to her symptoms. Linda had taken no medication other than the melatonin and the over-the-counter sleeping pills, which she'd run out of a week ago. She drank no alcohol and denied using any recreational drugs. Linda had stopped drinking all caffeinated beverages when the insomnia began several weeks ago. Her love life was not the greatest and she readily admitted, "That could be the whole problem."

When the psychiatrist asked her about any previous psychiatric treatment, Linda said she'd seen a psychiatrist four or five years ago in a different city. Her words trailed off, and there was a pregnant pause in the conversation, which had been flowing smoothly up until then. "Why did you seek help then, Linda?" Linda then more or less "confessed" about an embarrassing habit she had for years: hair pulling. She sheepishly took off a wig, which the psychiatrist hadn't even realized was a wig until that moment. The psychiatrist tried not to look stunned. Linda's face had not been strikingly beautiful, but she was undeniably pretty. Now, all of a sudden, she looked like a Buddhist monk. Linda quickly explained. "I shaved my head; I didn't pull all those out, but I had to shave it, or else I would have pulled them all out." Her parents, she said, had taken her to some sort of counselor for this problem when she was a child. Linda couldn't remember how old she was or much of anything about this counseling; "I was real young." Through grade school and high school, her hair pulling and plucking would come and go, and she could usually cover it up with the rest of her hair whenever there was a bald spot. Nobody ever noticed when she'd pull out the hair on her arms.

"Four or five years ago, it got really bad—the worst it had ever been—and I had to get some professional help." A psychiatrist then put her on an antidepressant, and a therapist had talked with Linda about her personal life and had helped her develop ways to control the hair-pulling compulsion. The compulsion had improved tremendously, and she stopped both therapy and the medication after she

had maintained a full head of hair for six months. But now, three years later, it was back. It had started up again several months ago, around the time her love life started to go sour and the depression began. She had "cleared" two bald spots the size of silver dollars before she decided to shave her head to stop herself. She then began working on her arms, her eyebrows, and her pubic hair.

Linda knew what she'd taken before, though she'd forgotten the dose. Her entire demeanor changed when the psychiatrist explained that this same medicine very well could work again to help both the depression and the trichotillomania. Linda seemed a bit embarrassed that it hadn't dawned on her to get back on the same medicine and that she hadn't come in for help before now. Sure enough, a combination of psychotherapy and several dose adjustments had Linda feeling good again and not pulling her hair.

Conversely, if a particular antidepressant did not help in the past, do not try it again. The exception to this rule, however, is if the medication, when tried before, was not given at the proper dose or for a long enough period of time. For example, sometimes patients admit that they previously decided on their own to discontinue their antidepressants due to side effects or lack of adequate response. Perhaps, however, their medicine would have been effective if they had lowered the dose a bit to reduce side effects or if they had raised the dose another notch or stayed on it for another week or two.

Fortunately, there are many effective medications available, and if a patient does not do well on one or prefers not to take it again, we can usually find another one (or a combination) that will help.

It is important to talk with your physician about everything that you and your family remember happening when you previously took a psychiatric medication. Often it is not a clear-cut, black or white "Yes, it worked great" or "No, it didn't help a bit." Often it is more of a gray area, "Well, it helped some but . . ." This information can be helpful. It may lead to using the same drug again, but in a higher dose or for a longer period of time, which could lead to a more robust response. Or it may lead to trying a chemically similar medication which is close enough to the previous one that it helps, but different enough that it works even better.

14

Chronological History

HOW LONG A SET OF SYMPTOMS has been present, its pattern over this time period, and whether or not there have been previous episodes of symptoms are vitally important data that you should discuss with your physician before starting antidepressant medication. It is important to establish, at the beginning, treatment goals and expectations that are realistic and attainable, and such a "chronological history" is a major predictor of what is a realistic and attainable outcome to aim for. Such a history is also a predictor of possible relapses or recurrences, thereby helping to determine whether the length of treatment should be relatively short (e.g., less than one year) or long (up to lifelong).

Let's start with the issue of how long a set of symptoms has been present. Generally speaking, the longer the symptoms have been present, the less likely that there will be a "full remission" (i.e., a total obliteration of symptoms). As an extreme example, consider somebody who has been "chronically depressed" (some patients say they have been depressed for their whole life

or for as long as they can remember). Such a patient will probably not do as well as somebody who did not develop any symptoms until the past couple of months. Your chronological
history will help give you and your doctor a realistic expectation of what outcome is attainable, and, consequently, the two
of you will be less likely to get upset, disappointed, and frustrated as a result of having set your hopes too high.

By the same token, you do not want to settle for less by
setting your hopes too low. It should be emphasized that in no
way should a history of chronic symptoms deter somebody
from seeking treatment with antidepressant medication. Some
of these patients can and do experience marked improvement.
And those who experience a partial (not full) recovery are still
quite thankful, frequently saying that at least they are better off
than what they used to be. Furthermore, through psychotherapy, they can learn new techniques to live with and manage
their remaining symptoms, and not let the symptoms ruin their
life.

In addition, there is another hopeful indicator for patients
whose symptoms began a long time ago: if the symptoms have
come and gone over the years, there is a better chance of a full
remission than if they have been there constantly the entire
time. This seems logical. After all, if your symptoms have gone
away on their own at times, then they ought to go away again at
some point, especially with some extra help from treatment.

Such a pattern of symptoms coming and going also has a
bearing on the length of treatment. If your symptoms have a
history of going away, then returning again at some later date,
they are likely to continue this pattern. Staying on antidepressant medication can prevent these recurrences, so long-term
treatment should be considered (see Chapter 37, "Prevention").

Your chronological history can also alert your doctor to the
possibility of another illness or additional symptoms that could
flare up during treatment. Knowing about these in advance can
help catch them early or even prevent them from happening.
Consider the following example and how treatment may have

gone smoother if a thorough chronological history had been obtained at the beginning.

🌿 Case Example

Overall, Susie was proud of her children and pretty proud of her parenting. She'd learned long ago that no child is perfect and that it is not always Mom's fault when a child isn't doing well. She was well beyond imposing blame on herself for her children's imperfections. Besides, the kids were doing fairly well right now. So when Susie was trying to figure out why she'd been feeling kind of blue lately, she rejected the "mother's guilt" theory. The children certainly weren't around anywhere near as much as they used to be, so the "empty nest" syndrome could be contributing, she thought to herself. She had taken a job to fill in some time and thought the work would be both fun and interesting. The pay wasn't great, but it wasn't bad either, and she had met some interesting people.

But Susie's enthusiasm for the job was waning. In fact, her enthusiasm for practically everything was waning. She continued to go to her usual activities but pretty much had to force herself to go. And when she went, the activities weren't as much fun as they used to be. She was tired and would find herself thinking, "I'd really rather be home in bed right now." At home, when she had the chance, she did go to bed and would put off until later those things that could wait. She knew something was wrong; she felt "blunted"—not only emotionally and physically but also mentally. Susie had always felt she was probably above average in intelligence—until now. Now she didn't feel as sharp mentally. She wasn't as witty or as quick in her thinking. She noticed at times that she would lose her train of thought and have to start over.

So Susie went to her doctor, who diagnosed depression and began her on an antidepressant. She also referred Susie to a psychologist, and psychological testing confirmed the diagnosis of depression. Susie began seeing the psychologist in individual therapy and took her antidepressant religiously. Two months and several dose increases later, not only was Susie still depressed, she was worse. Her doctor referred her to a psychiatrist, who agreed with the diagnosis. The psychiatrist also agreed with how Susie's treatment had been managed so far: it had been appropriate treatment, it just hadn't worked. The psychiatrist switched Susie to another antidepressant and encouraged her to continue her psychotherapy with the psychologist. He worked closely with Susie over the next several weeks, increasing the dose and explaining to her what he was doing and why.

Finally, Susie's depression began to lift. The first thing she noticed was the energy creeping back into her body, and she could almost physically feel her sense of humor returning. Once the logjam began to break, Susie got unstuck very quickly. Within a few days, Susie felt good again. Gone was the empty feeling of nothingness; back was her old enthusiasm. Gone went the dull thinking and hermitlike behavior; back came her wit, extroversion, and confidence. Susie couldn't believe the contrast. "Wow, what a 180! That drug is a miracle drug!"

Unfortunately, though, Susie overshot the mark and began feeling too good. She laughed hysterically at things that weren't that funny. She was downright giddy. She never seemed to run low on energy. To the contrary, she was full of get-up-and-go. Those who got in her way better look out. She only slept a few hours a night, then would wake up "raring to go." Her mind was speeding, and so was her speech. You couldn't shut her up. Her friends and coworkers became concerned. In fact, they wondered if she was taking speed. Some bold friends verbalized their concern to Susie, who just laughed them off. "I'm feeling good again and I'm going to enjoy it. I'm not taking anything. I don't need my antidepressant or anything anymore!" They alerted Susie's psychiatrist, who also tried to talk to her, but to no avail. She wouldn't even return to see him anymore. "I don't need any dinky-shrinky anymore; I'm fine." Not too much later, Susie was fired for being rude with clients and insubordinate with her supervisor. She then spent all the money she made at work on new clothes—some of them pretty outlandish.

Eventually, Susie became so out of control that she required hospitalization, where she was diagnosed as being in a manic episode. She had bipolar disorder (what used to be called manic-depressive

WARNING SIGNS OF A MANIC EPISODE

A. Abnormally and persistently elevated, expansive, or irritable mood
B. During this mood disturbance, such symptoms as:
    1. Inflated self-esteem or grandiosity
    2. Decreased need for sleep (i.e., feels rested after only three hours of sleep)
    3. More talkative than usual
    4. Racing thoughts
    5. Distractibility
    6. Significant increase in activities, or agitation
    7. Excessive activities that are pleasurable but have a high risk for negative consequences (e.g., buying sprees, sexual indiscretions, foolish business investments)

Adapted from the American Psychiatric Association's *Diagnostic and Statistical Manual of Mental Disorders*, Fourth Edition.

illness), and the antidepressant had not only brought her out of her depression, it also triggered a manic episode.

During Susie's first appointment, a more careful, thorough evaluation of her chronological history would have alerted Susie's psychiatrist to this possibility. When she was eighteen, Susie had experienced a similar episode of being "on a high" and had to drop out of school. It wasn't diagnosed or treated back then and had subsided on its own. Had Susie's psychiatrist known about her previous episode, this manic episode may have been prevented, or at least nipped in the bud.

Susie recovered nicely from the manic episode with lithium treatment, but they wouldn't hire her back at work. It took her months to get over the embarrassment and humiliation she felt over some of the things she

*said and did when she was manic. Eventually, she made a full recovery,
and Susie has had no further manic or depressive episodes. She has been
on lithium for nine years now.*

The presence of a manic episode in one's chronological
history is a red flag for the psychiatrist treating that patient.
Once someone has had a confirmed manic episode, he has
bipolar disorder, and a depression that comes from bipolar
disorder is a horse of a different color than a depression in
someone who has never had a manic episode. The treatment
approach for an episode of depression in a bipolar patient is
usually different, since there is a possibility that an
antidepressant can trigger a manic episode.

Similarly, if symptoms of a manic episode occur during
antidepressant treatment, the patient's physician should be
notified promptly. Therefore, people taking antidepressants, and
their families, should be aware of bipolar disorder and the signs
and symptoms of a manic episode.

15

Genetic Factors

GENETIC FACTORS FREQUENTLY CONTRIBUTE to the appearance of depressive, obsessive-compulsive, panic, or attention-deficit/hyperactivity symptoms in an individual. If you have a relative who has had symptoms similar to yours, and he or she has had a positive response to a certain medication, then that medication would be a good drug for you to try first. Some psychiatrists believe that, just as an illness can run in a family, a genetic responsivity to a certain medicine can run in a family too.

 CASE EXAMPLE

> *John stopped drinking again, and again he and the others hoped it would be for good. How many times had he stopped before—ten or fifteen? Maybe twenty? Enough times that he was "easy pickin's" for the cynics in his neighborhood: "John? Quit for good? Riiight!" Then they would all get a good laugh (at John's expense).*
>
> *But this time maybe it would be different. This time John and his*

wife had a different plan. She had learned of a fairly new treatment idea called a dual diagnosis program, geared for people who had not only a chemical dependency or alcoholism diagnosis but also a second, coexisting diagnosis. She was convinced that John had something more than just pure alcoholism: Anxiety? Depression? Both? Something else? She didn't know for sure what it was he had, but he had something *else going on, and if it could be fixed, then maybe John could stay on the wagon.*

She had seen it happen so often, she could predict the pattern: After a particular bad episode, John would quit drinking and attend AA for a while, but sooner or later, she'd notice him looking more nervous, jittery, and on edge. She knew it wasn't withdrawal from the alcohol, which he'd stopped several weeks earlier. John would get more negative and irritable, worried about his job and their finances, and gripe about every dime she'd spent. He didn't want to go out and do things anymore and lost his sense of humor. He didn't always sleep very well, and occasionally he mentioned feeling tense or complained of muscle tension in his neck and shoulders. He sure looked tense to her. She was sure one *of the reasons John would start drinking again was to "self-medicate," and she hoped the dual diagnosis program would eliminate his need to do this. She knew John was a good person and really wanted to stay dry, and she hoped that "getting his nerves under control" would help him stay sober and* improve *his quality of life.*

John was skeptical but went to the appointment she had scheduled for him. He admitted to the psychiatrist that he'd been a worrier and a nervous person "as far back as I can remember," but added, "To be honest, I don't think that's why I drink. I've been through that thing before where you try to find a reason why you drink, something to blame it on. There's a thousand things I could blame it on, but that's not the answer. I just need to keep going to [AA] meetings and working the Steps." The psychiatrist, somewhat to John's surprise, said she heartily agreed, although she had a few things she wanted to add. "Maybe you've got more than just alcoholism going on, John. It could be like what my vet said when my dog was itching so bad: 'Maybe it's fleas and lice.' Let's take a look at your nervousness."

The doctor proceeded with gathering a thorough history, performed a brief physical examination, and eventually reached a conclusion. "John, I don't think you have two diagnoses. I think you have three: alcoholism, anxiety, and depression." John had told the psychiatrist about his brother in California, who'd had similar problems in the past but was doing quite well currently. The psychiatrist then asked John if he would mind calling his brother and asking if his brother had taken any medicine and, if so, which one, and did it help? John said he would, but he thought it was a moot point because "I ain't takin' any tranquilizer or antidepressant or nerve pill or nothin'."

At the next appointment, John reported that his brother had, indeed, taken a medicine. It was an antidepressant, and his brother thought it had helped immensely and was still taking it. Not only that, John also learned that their uncle was taking the same antidepressant, and the uncle also thought it had made a difference in his life. Nevertheless, John said, "I ain't takin' it. I've gone to chemicals too many times. I've tried escaping into the bottle. I'm chemically dependent. I need to stay away from drugs, not start a new one!"

The psychiatrist emphatically supported John's intent and said she respected John's resolve, but (like before) she had a few things she wanted to add. "The antidepressants are different, John. They work on different chemicals in the brain than alcohol, tranquilizers, or street drugs. They are not addicting. They won't make you high. They are not an escape or a cop-out, but they can stabilize your mood and lessen your anxiety. There might be something genetic going on in your family—something you and your brother and your uncle all inherited. This medicine is not going to be a magic pill that makes you live happily ever after, but it could act as an ally to the Twelve Steps and the AA meetings. It could improve the quality of your life, not to mention your wife's." They discussed the issue for about ten more minutes. John felt the psychiatrist meant well, but he politely declined treatment with medication and left.

A few years later John showed up at the psychiatrist's office again. He'd had two more relapses with alcohol and was separated

*from his wife. "Doctor, I'm ready to try that medicine. My brother
is still doing great, and I keep messing up."*

Genetic factors can also be relevant diagnostically. If you
have a family history of bipolar disorder, then you are statisti-
cally more likely to have bipolar disorder than the Average Joe.
The same is true for panic disorder, obsessive-compulsive disorder, and attention-deficit/hyperactivity disorder. In the event
you do have a positive family history, you should be aware of
the signs and symptoms of the disorder that runs in your family.
Furthermore, you and your doctor should spend extra time
looking for that disorder in you, and you both should recognize
its signs and symptoms if it crops up in the future.

16

The Truth, the Whole Truth, and Nothing but the Truth

THERE MAY BE SOME THINGS about which you feel guilty, embarrassed, or ashamed. Naturally, we humans like to keep these things private. Nevertheless, it is important that your doctor knows about these things, for they could make a difference in how successful your treatment is. Consider the following example.

🌿 CASE EXAMPLE

Elizabeth was smartly dressed and pretty. Her mostly white hair was attractively coiffured and her jewelry simple yet elegant. Her husband was seated in the waiting room. His snow-white hair and mustache were neatly trimmed and his three-piece suit was nicely tailored. The psychiatrist's assumption that they were financially comfortable was more or less confirmed later by occasional comments that Elizabeth made about "the country club," "the Cadillac," and "our Florida place."

Elizabeth would also have been a good case example to demon-

strate the old saying "money can't buy happiness," for Elizabeth was depressed, as depressed as they come. She had walked into the office with a confident, stately air about her, but in five minutes her composure was out the window. She didn't just cry; her sobs were gut-wrenching. She was in pain. She went on to describe a constellation of symptoms that was a textbook description of depression and that had just started this year. She was in good health and was on no medication. She had never seen a psychiatrist before and had never taken any kind of tranquilizer or antidepressant. There was an aunt who had been in a "state hospital for the insane" decades ago, but no other psychiatric illness in the family. She drank alcohol and admitted she had been drinking too much the past year. "It was the only way I could get to sleep, Doctor."

Her husband later confirmed her history. She had never had a drinking problem before, but now he was quite concerned about her alcohol consumption. It had grown from the usual one cocktail before dinner to two cocktails before dinner plus "God knows how many after dinner." She often slurred by the time they went to bed. In the past two months, he noticed she'd already had a few by the time he came home from the office, and he had insisted that she come to this appointment.

The psychiatrist determined that she was not in danger of any serious alcohol withdrawal symptoms or DTs if she quit drinking abruptly, then asked her to completely abstain from alcohol. Elizabeth was given some medicine to help her come off the alcohol and to sleep better over the next week. At the next appointment, both Elizabeth and her husband confirmed that she had not had a drop to drink in the interim.

Elizabeth's depression remained the same. The second session consisted primarily of exploring the possible factors that could have contributed to this depression, and discussing antidepressant medications. Elizabeth was started on an antidepressant. In the next few sessions, the psychiatrist explained more about the medicine, and they talked more about the possible contributing factors. There wasn't much to talk about, though, because Elizabeth felt she really was a "very lucky woman who has everything."

Over the next few weeks, Elizabeth continued to take her an-

tidepressant and remained abstinent from alcohol. By the fifth session, Elizabeth was no better. It was during that session that she confided to her psychiatrist that she thought she was guilty of murder. She went on to explain how, decades ago, she had been a chaperon on a hayride where one of the youths tragically fell off the wagon and was crushed to death. Her guilt and grief had been horrendous after the accident, even though the youth's family had repeatedly reassured her that they did not hold her responsible in the least. Elizabeth said she thought she had worked her way through the guilt and grief over the next few years, and said she'd barely even thought about it for the past twenty years. Nobody in her community had even mentioned it in about ten years. But the event reappeared in her head this past year, and Elizabeth wondered if her current depression was God's way of punishing her for her negligence on the hayride.

Elizabeth wept uncontrollably as she told her story, the sobs coming from deep within her. She said she'd hoped she wouldn't have to tell anybody about this, to "reopen Pandora's box." She hadn't told her husband or anybody, but the thoughts were there every day. "I think that is why I'm depressed, Doctor. I'd rather be dead. In fact, I wish I was dead. I deserve to die for what I did to that poor child. I deserve to die and to go to hell, but God is keeping me alive and keeping me alive for a reason. I'm in hell now. God's got me in hell."

It had been quite difficult for Elizabeth to "spill her guts" about this to someone else. Her "confession" moved the psychotherapy to a higher plane, a deeper, more meaningful level, than it had been on before. Interestingly, her revelation also had a bearing on the pharmacological aspect of her treatment, and a second medicine was added to her antidepressant. Elizabeth recovered fully from her depression.

Most cases are not as dramatic as Elizabeth's, but revealing a very personal issue like this can be a turning point in a patient's recovery. Such an extremely private, personal issue may be a key factor in *causing* the illness in the first place, or it may be more a *manifestation* of the illness than a cause (see Chapter 33, "Cause and Effect"). In either case, it is important that your doctor know about it. Such an emotionally laden issue certainly warrants discussion.

Personal "secrets" and facts about oneself that are "hidden away in a closet" are commonly seen in the illnesses treated by the antidepressants. Low self-esteem, guilt, and shame are part and parcel of depression, and people just don't go around broadcasting these aspects of themselves, or things they have done, that they are not very proud of. People with OCD are often embarrassed or ashamed of the thoughts that repetitively intrude into their mind and/or the rituals that they are compelled to do. People with eating disorders are notorious for keeping their behaviors secret from family and friends. This being the nature of the beast to begin with, the natural tendency is to continue to keep this information hidden. However, it is important to remember that these phenomena are part of the illness. For treatment purposes, think of there being a "healthy part" of you and an "unhealthy part" of you. The healthy part forms this alliance with the treating physician and tells it all: "the whole truth and nothing but the truth."

It is not easy to do this. It takes humility and courage to bare one's soul, but it is worth it.

17

Alcohol, Caffeine, and Recreational Drugs, Part I

THE PRESCRIBING PHYSICIAN needs to know *accurately* to what extent you are using alcohol, caffeine, and recreational drugs ("substances"). These substances really muddy the water when trying to do the initial evaluation and decide how much the symptoms are a direct result of the primary psychiatric illness versus how much they are a (direct or indirect) result of the substance. Fluctuations of blood and brain levels of alcohol, for example, can cause insomnia, nervousness, restlessness, agitation, shakiness, tremors, irritability, rapid heartbeat and palpitations, rapid breathing, excessive perspiration, dilated pupils, bad dreams, confusion, light-headedness, and moodiness. Because of this, experienced specialists in the chemical dependency field often wait until after an alcoholic is detoxified before deciding to treat him or her for depression or a primary anxiety disorder. It is now well known that many alcoholics have a coexisting but separate psychiatric illness in addition to their alcoholism (a "dual diagnosis"). The symptoms of their nonalcohol-related depression or anxiety don't disappear after detoxification is complete, and they need treatment for *both* their diagnoses. But not uncommonly, the symptoms of depression or anxiety will be much better (if not gone) after detoxification is complete. Chris's case is a good example of this.

🌿 CASE EXAMPLE

For years, Chris had ignored his then-wife's and friends' pleas to get a routine checkup with a doctor. They cited high blood pressure, prostate cancer, and rectal cancer as examples of dangerous illnesses that can be caught early by such an examination, if he would only get one. Chris was a strong and hardy soul, was in decent physical shape, and could be pretty stubborn and oppositional when others tried to give him advice. In the past ten years, he'd seen his doctor only twice, and both times not until he was really sick. Chris was proud of his overall healthiness. So it was no small thing when Chris made an appointment to see the doctor, especially when he was seeking help for depression and his nerves. Macho Chris, asking for help?! Something really had to be wrong.

Something really was wrong. Chris had been moody and irritable before, but not like this. He'd never snapped at people at the office before, but now it was becoming almost a daily thing. He admitted to his buddies at work that he wasn't happy, and he hadn't been really happy since way before his divorce. He was tense and shaky, couldn't wait until he got off work, which is when he went to his favorite watering hole and had a couple of drinks. He couldn't sleep through the night without waking up, and sometimes he couldn't fall back to sleep. Chris told his doctor about his problems and asked, "So do I have anxiety or depression, or what, Doc? What kind of a psycho am I? Can you give me an antidepressant or a tranquilizer or something? How about a sleeping pill? I really could use some sleep."

Chris's doctor was cautious in choosing his words. "I don't know for sure what you've got, Chris. Let me ask you some more questions and let's run some tests, then I'll have a better idea." Chris's doctor happened to be privy to some inside information about Chris. He'd been the family's doctor for over twenty years and had taken care of all of the children and Chris's ex-wife. Even before the divorce, Chris's wife had mentioned the alcohol issue to the doctor. Remembering this, the doctor asked Chris some routine doctor-type questions, then asked Chris how much alcohol he drank. Chris did a good job of being vague in his answer and making it sound minimal. They finished up, the doctor ordered some tests, then scheduled Chris for an appointment the following week.

The tests came back okay, including Chris's liver tests (which the doctor had been most concerned about). The doctor told Chris this good news and then told Chris what he had heard over the years about Chris's drinking and how he was suspicious that the alcohol may be a significant contributor to Chris's current symptoms. "How much do you drink, really, Chris?" Chris acknowledged that he drank every day—though rarely enough to get a "buzz." Sometimes, he admitted, he got a buzz when he hadn't really meant to, but he rarely got really drunk—"only once or twice per year."

They met a few more times over the next few months, and at the doctor's suggestion, Chris stopped drinking entirely. The doctor gave Chris some medicine for the first couple of weeks to help him sleep, then said, "Okay, Chris, this is the acid test. We're going to wean you off this medicine and see how you do au naturel: no alcohol, no tranquilizers, no sleeping pill, no antidepressant. No drugs, period. You ready?"

Chris was ready and gave it a try. His symptoms, which had already improved some after he stopped drinking, continued to improve. In a few weeks, Chris's anxiety and depression were gone. He never needed an antidepressant.

Everybody knows how alcohol can affect the liver, but not many people know that it harms the brain more often than it harms the liver.

Caffeine can also complicate the picture when trying to do an initial evaluation. Caffeine can mimic the symptoms of panic and anxiety. The following case illustrates this.

❧ Case Example

Sandra was brought to the crisis center by her sister and some friends. She asked if she could be "put on Prozac or something for my nerves."

She was a recently divorced mother who had been depressed ever since her marriage began to deteriorate. She had taken a decent-paying night shift job to help with the finances, and her mother baby-sat for the children at night. She slept (or tried to sleep) during the day when the children were at school and when she was finished with her tasks of chauffeuring, grocery shopping, housecleaning, etc. Her friends and family thought she was doing okay and initially did not think that her depression was out of proportion to what she was going through. However, after a while, she began looking more tired and haggard. She developed a tremor and admitted that she felt shaky and nervous. She was jumpy, startled easily, and began snapping at the children. She attributed this to "what I'm going through" and the fact that "I've not been sleeping much." Indeed, she was constantly on the go and burning the candle at both ends, attending to all her parental responsibilities.

Eventually, her sister and friends made her come in for an evaluation because she had become "so wired, strung out, and scatter-brained"—not her usual self. The sister had taken Prozac and improved, and thought it might help Sandra too.

The first thing the crisis worker did when talking with Sandra alone was to subtly lead the conversation around to the subject of Sandra's misery and how bad it was. The social worker needed to know how much pain Sandra was in, if Sandra had recently felt as if she'd rather be dead, if Sandra had recently had any thoughts about suicide, about abandoning her children or about killing them. She asked if Sandra had physically injured or struck them in any way. Sandra seemed a little put off by the innuendo and the way the conversation was flowing, but she quickly understood when the crisis worker explained that a top priority was to ensure that nobody got hurt. That made sense to Sandra, and she respected the crisis worker's ethic of checking this out first.

They then got down to doing a more thorough assessment. There appeared to be a possible genetic tendency in the family: Sandra's mother and uncle had also had problems, though they had never been treated, as Sandra's sister had been. There was no history of any previous episodes or treatment, and Sandra was in good health, as far as she knew. She'd never had any thyroid problems. She was on no other medicines (including over-the-counter medicines), didn't drink any alcohol, and had never once taken any recreational drugs. Then they got to caffeine. Sandra admitted that she had been drinking several cups of coffee upon arising to help her wake up when the children got home from school, then periodically drank more coffee and caffeinated beverages throughout the evening to "help keep me going" and on the job from 11:00 P.M. to 7:00 A.M. "to keep me awake."

While not ignoring all the stress she was under and the internal pain she was feeling, part of the treatment strategy (before beginning any medication) was to help her "decaffeinate" from her daily consumption of ten to sixteen cups of coffee (or its equivalent). Not surprisingly, she improved without needing any prescription antidepressants.

Both "caffeinism" (what Sandra had) and caffeine withdrawal symptoms (including fatigue, headache, and excessive sleep) can cause psychiatric symptoms. Before we blame stress or chemical imbalances in the brain for causing all the problems, do not forget caffeine. Imagine how many cups of coffee are consumed every day in the United States.

Using drugs for "recreation" is not a healthful thing to do to begin with, but it certainly has no place at all, and should be completely avoided, when someone is suffering from a psychiatric disorder. Studies have shown that marijuana usage can worsen depression. Cocaine, "uppers," and diet pills can worsen or mimic anxiety and panic, and coming off of them can cause depression. The effects of, and withdrawal from, "downers" are similar to those of alcohol, causing a variety of psychiatric symptoms that are difficult to distinguish from the symptoms of a primary psychiatric illness. Psychedelic drugs and hallucinogens put the same brain chemicals *out* of balance that psychiatrists try to put back *into* balance.

All it takes is a little common sense to figure out that street drugs, caffeine, and alcohol can all have a significant effect on one's body. It is essential for your physician to know about your use of these before he or she prescribes any antidepressant.

What to Expect

18

The Therapeutic Alliance, Part II: Working Together

JUST AS YOU NEED TO BE COMPLETELY open and honest with your physician, so does your physician need to be open and honest with you. It goes both ways. Once your doctor has a diagnosis and treatment plan in mind, he or she should share it with you. People who develop these disorders are understandably anxious about what is happening to them and what the future holds for them. Your doctor should alleviate this anxiety by giving you a basic explanation about the illness in general and about your individually tailored treatment plan. Without this knowledge, your anxiety could needlessly continue and could impede or delay your recovery.

It is reassuring to hear from an expert that he knows what is wrong and can help. Knowing that your doctor listened to you and understands your case should instill faith in your doctor, and learning hard facts should instill hope for your recovery. Hope, faith, and confidence in both the doctor and the treatment plan are powerful, nonpharmacological contributors to the healing process. If a doctor plunges into treatment without explaining to you what he is doing and why, your recovery will not go as smoothly as it should, even if the treatment is correct. Furthermore, a patient with unanswered questions and significant anxiety about a medication is less likely to take that medication as directed (which, of course, decreases the odds of improvement).

If you are lucky, after an antidepressant is first started, you will have a 100 percent response on the first try. Otherwise, you will need to report back to your doctor about what has happened (no response, partial response, side effects, or whatever). Then, by hearing these reports, your physician can make the necessary adjustments to meet your particular needs, all the while explaining what he is doing. This continuing dialogue is essential to successful treatment. Your reports to your doctor should not be of a complaining or accusatory nature (e.g., about how treatment is not working or how he has not done his job), but should be a frank and matter-of-fact description of what specifically is still wrong. Your physician's response should not be one of a condescending or "don't bother me" nature, but should likewise be frank and matter-of-fact. Both of you should be comfortable enough with each other to "call a spade a spade." You tell it like it is, your doctor tweaks the dose, adjusts the timing, or changes the medication, and together you discuss what you hope to see. This ongoing approach will not leave you hanging with an inadequate response or troublesome side effects, not knowing what to do next. Such a team approach to pharmacological management enables the necessary adjustments to be made, so that the proper dose of the proper medication reaches your brain. And, along the way, it builds the bonds of the doctor-patient relationship and bolsters each other's resolve to carry on the fight against the illness.

Chapters 19 to 26 contain basic information about what to expect when taking an antidepressant and may serve as a springboard for discussions with your physician about your particular case.

19

Aesop's Tortoise

WHEN YOU TAKE MEDICATION for an upset stomach, a headache, an asthma attack, pain, tranquilization, insomnia, or any number of physical symptoms, you expect it to kick in within minutes, or at least within an hour, and it usually does. Not so with the antidepressants, though, which take an average of three or four weeks before they really start kicking in. And it is important to note that this three or four weeks starts from when the proper dose of the proper medication was begun, not from when the very first dose of the medication was taken.

Some people ("rapid responders") are lucky and improve within the first week or two. Some, though, are on the other end of the bell-shaped curve, taking six weeks or longer. But most people will improve, if they are going to improve on that dose, within three or four weeks of beginning that dose. However, be forewarned that in the case of someone who requires several dosage changes and/or medication changes, it may be months (or, on occasion, a few years) before improvement is noted. Therefore, it is extremely important for you to know from the very start that the course of your recovery could seem like the course of a marathon runner: unbelievably long.

🌿 CASE EXAMPLE

Lori had her first panic attack about a month after moving to a new state. Within minutes her heart was racing and pounding, and she felt a tightness in her chest. She was light-headed, and everything around her had a stilted, sort of imaginary look to it. "I felt as if I was watching a movie," she said later. She rushed to a walk-in, "quick-care" medical clinic located close to her neighborhood, where she was assessed, treated, and then referred to a young family physician who was just starting her practice. The first attack had resolved completely, but each subsequent day, she'd experienced a "pressure" or "full feeling" in her head, fatigue, dizziness, and anxiety. The tranquilizers she'd received from the clinic helped the anxiety, but she still didn't feel right. Furthermore, several times a week she'd have a flare-up of the panic and again experience the pounding heart, pressure in her chest, shortness of breath, shaking, "awkward" stomach, feeling of detachment, and a hot/flushed feeling. She was afraid of "losing control," or going insane and doing something crazy (though she didn't know what it was she might do). She began awakening every morning with the thought "What's wrong with me?" and with the fear of having a day full of anxiety. During the day, she became preoccupied with her symptoms and her fears, wondering if she'd ever have a normal life again.

Her new physician explained panic disorder to her, and Lori felt reassured that somebody knew what was wrong and that it was fixable. Nevertheless, Lori was getting progressively more frightened of having another panic attack and began dreading it every time she had to leave her new home. Twice she called in sick to work, and she began cutting classes. The young physician added an antidepressant to the tranquilizer and explained to Lori that it would not *work quickly, but in the meantime, she would like Lori to see a psychologist.*

Lori saw the psychologist and was soon given some relaxation exercises and techniques to practice, as well as a book to read. She learned how catastrophizing contributes to panic, and learned how to use the techniques of thought stopping and cognitive restructuring. She listened to a few tapes at home and practiced her homework assignments. Lori and her psychologist discussed her anxiety about the move, her career uncertainty, stress she was experiencing in school, and some conflicts she was having with her boyfriend. Lori made herself go to work and school, even when she didn't feel like it.

Four weeks later Lori was better. She now felt confident that she was in control, even when some of the panic symptoms were there. She was determined not to let the symptoms control her. A month later she felt back to normal.

Lori's response was not overnight, but it was right on schedule for how fast an antidepressant works (especially when combined with appropriate psychotherapy). Lori was lucky to have responded to the first medicine and to the first dose she ever tried. Dorothy's case is more typical.

✿ Case Example

Dorothy was no stranger to depression, having required hospital- ization for a severe depression around the time of her menopause in the 1970s. She recovered well, however, and had really enjoyed herself the past twenty years. "I've been to hell (excuse the French)," she was known for saying, "and now I appreciate God's wonders more than I did before my trip." She had become an avid bird-watcher and was so spunky that sometimes she left the others (most of them younger than she) in the dust as she scurried through the fields and woods. A more doting, loving grandmother did not exist; until she got depressed again, that is.

It started with insomnia, and a decrease in her appetite soon followed. She lost ten pounds. Her doctor found nothing physically wrong with her. Her vim and vigor died, and her personality went flat. It was springtime and the warblers came and went, but she didn't go birding once. She said she couldn't care less. She didn't even enjoy being around her grandchildren anymore. Dorothy reluctantly went to the psychiatrist when her family insisted, stating she didn't think it mattered because her life was about over anyway. She confided to her psychiatrist that she had been praying for God to take her—that she was ready. She denied being suicidal at all—"I'd never do that. My father did that, and I'd never do that to my family. Besides, it's a sin."

Her psychiatrist began seeing her weekly for psychotherapy and began her on what he hoped was the same medicine that she had taken twenty years ago (Dorothy couldn't remember its name for sure). She began sleeping better within a few days, but it still was not a restful sleep. Four weeks later she said she was "pretty good." When pressed to estimate how much *better she was feeling, she guessed she was "maybe 50 percent back." She didn't look "50 percent back" to her psychiatrist, even though he had never seen her before she got depressed and thereby did not know how she looked normally. He knew how she looked now—flat as a pancake.*

After a few more weeks, Dorothy admitted she was still only "about 50 percent," and the psychiatrist upped her dose. She then felt overmedicated, drugged and "fuzzy-headed," but she continued the higher dosage like a trouper, hoping her head would clear with time. It didn't. Her dose was lowered back down, and she said she felt better. However, she still looked depressed, and she admitted she was nowhere near being her usual self.

Over the next four months, Dorothy and her psychiatrist continued to meet weekly. They talked about much more than her medication, since neither of them believed that the medicine could "do it all." They stopped the first antidepressant and tried a second one. At first, it didn't do anything. They upped the dose and she felt a little better. They upped it again and she began feeling nauseated, so they lowered it again, but she seemed to plateau there, so they upped it again—but not as much.

A few weeks later her psychiatrist thought Dorothy looked a little brighter and had a bit more spring in her step as she walked from the waiting room into the office. Sure enough, Dorothy acknowledged she was "feeling human" again. She was not just making herself *eat and go places, she was beginning to enjoy her food and activities again. The good days were outnumbering the bad days. However, most nights she still wasn't sleeping straight through the night, and she was still having some bad days. They upped the dose again and waited for the nausea to happen again. It did happen, but then went away.*

Within four weeks, Dorothy was sleeping well again. She looked like a new person to her psychiatrist, and she beamed when describing her plans to take her granddaughter to some wetlands to see the sandhill cranes drop in for a night's rest while on their way South. A total of six months had passed.

Dorothy's case is fairly typical. Many people need to try more than one drug and require several dosage adjustments before they receive a full response to an antidepressant. Others, however, take even *longer* than Dorothy.

🌿 CASE EXAMPLE

Candy was a dream nurse—the kind all doctors and hospital administrators dream about having. Conscientious to the nth degree, she didn't let anything slip through the cracks. She had been promoted up the chain of command to the rank of head nurse, and she still received rave reviews from her patients, even though she now spent hours doing administrative work in addition to patient care. One of the secrets to her success, in addition to her strong work ethic, was the fact that she worked extra hours—coming in to work early and leaving work late. Candy didn't mind that she was not getting paid for this extra time; she just wanted to make sure "the job was done right."

One year she began staying later than usual, and then she occasionally even returned to work in the middle of her drive home. Others began saying things to her about her working too hard, and a few friends became concerned about her. Enough is enough, and this was too much—even for Candy!

It turned out that Candy could not let go of the thought that maybe, somehow, she had accidentally made an error at work and somebody might die or suffer a serious injury because of her error. At first, she was staying later than usual in order to double- and triple-check IV sites, infusions, and medication orders. As her illness worsened, she had to return to the hospital to check them yet again, after she had already triple-checked them before she left. The list of what she had to check grew, and soon she was checking nonmedical items too, such as the work schedule, to ensure she'd not left any shift uncovered, and the report tape, to ensure nothing had been accidentally left off the report to the next shift. Eventually, she ended up seeing a psychiatrist and a therapist.

While Candy's therapist worked with her on the nonpharmacological techniques she could use to combat her compulsions, the psychiatrist managed the medication component of her treatment. She'd been a perfectionist for years and had always had a few quirks: all the clothes in her closet and all the silverware in the drawer had to be arranged "just so," and whenever she touched a sharp object, she had to silently count to seven. But she had never been this bad before and had never received treatment. Though Candy's mother was also described as being similarly obsessive-compulsive, she had never been treated either. Candy discussed the options with her psychiatrist, then started taking an antidepressant.

To make a long story short, Candy was tried on a total of seven medicines (some of them in combination with each other). At one point, she was unable to work, and on another occasion, she became so despondent that hospitalization was required. Finally, after four years of treatment, Candy was okay again. She was still fairly perfectionistic, but not neurotically so, and she was able to go home at quitting time and enjoy a balanced life. She was not totally free of all rituals, but the remaining ones were minor and did not control her life.

Candy's case history, like Lori's, is also atypical—though hers is on the other end of the spectrum. Most people do not take four years to get better. Though Candy's case is an extreme example, it helps emphasize the point that treatment with the antidepressants can take a long time.

. . .

Nobody knows why it takes so long for the antidepressants to work. As described in Chapter 1, researchers believe the effectiveness of the antidepressants is somehow related to their activity around and in the synapse: their action on the neurotransmitters and the receptors on the nerve endings. With the very first dose, your medicine will begin the process of bathing these nerve endings. Although you will probably feel nothing, a fundamental transformation is beginning to occur around, on the surfaces of, and inside these nerves. This transformation moves slowly, like the tortoise in Aesop's famous fable, requiring several weeks of cumulative action before you will notice significant improvement. Don't give up . . . remember who won the race with the hare.

That it takes so long for these medications to begin working is unfortunate, but this time can be well spent. Most patients who are waiting for the benefits of an antidepressant to kick in will also benefit from counseling or psychotherapy. It does not help to just sit there getting impatient. Rather than waiting passively for the medicine to "do it all," you can be actively doing those nonpharmacological things you need to do to contribute to your improvement. Psychotherapy, like medication, takes time to work, and the odds of improvement are better if you use both treatment modalities simultaneously (see Chapter 34, "Psychotherapy").

With the guidance of your therapist, and on your own, work on achieving "a balance" to your life. Be sure that you eat nutritiously every day or, if you are simply unable to do so, maintain your nutrition by ingesting enough vitamins and food supplements to compensate. Exercise regularly. Even though you may not feel like exercising, make yourself do it. Research has documented that exercise has a therapeutic, antidepressant effect. Work, too, is therapy. Whether you get paid for it or are doing it voluntarily, spend at least some time doing some work. Be productive, creative. Contribute. Accomplish something. Also find some time for play. Even though your previous "play" activities may not bring you the pleasure they used to, at least go through the motions. Sooner or later, you will begin to enjoy them again, and having fun can help recharge your batteries. Last but not least, don't lose contact with your spirituality. Not uncommonly, when in the throes of a psychiatric illness, people lose faith or distance themselves from their spiritual life. They may feel abandoned or rejected by their God, or they may abandon or reject their God. Of all times, this is *the time* to nurture your religion and faith, not to detach.

And when you are not working on finding and maintaining the proper balance for your life, or are not in a psychotherapy session or working on any psychotherapy homework, at least keep busy doing something. When you are not busy, your inactivity becomes the fertile soil in which psychiatric symptoms thrive. Doing "nothing" allows negative thoughts and feelings to flourish and to crowd out positive and constructive thoughts and feelings (like weeds taking over a garden). On the contrary, being busy keeps your mind focused on something else, which helps prevent these negative thoughts and feelings from popping up and taking over. Don't just sit in a chair or lie in bed and do nothing.

Some patients make the mistake of passively waiting for the medicine to kick in. This is a big mistake. Along with unilaterally adjusting one's own dosage, it is the other most common mistake leading to treatment failure. Even when you don't feel like it, do your usual daily routine or make yourself do *something*. Keep yourself occupied until you are okay again ("fake it till you make it"). The act of being active actually works in conjunction with the medicine to speed your recovery.

20

Which Antidepressant
Is "the Best"? Finding
the Right Medicine

N O ONE PSYCHIATRIC MEDICINE is "the best." No one medicine is going to work for everybody. Everyone is different.
Some people will improve with drug A and not with drug B,
and others will improve with drug B and not with drug A. It all
boils down to getting the best match between an individual's
unique body chemistry and the pharmacological action of an
individual drug.

Finding the medicine that best matches your unique body
chemistry is not as difficult as it may seem. Medication options
are more or less ranked and selected based on the information
you reveal about yourself (see "What to Say to the Doctor,"
Chapters 9 to 17). Previous response (or nonresponse) to a particular medicine is tremendously important. Similarly, previous
side effects (or lack of side effects) to a particular medicine help
narrow down the options. Also important are the specific target
symptoms and signs from which you need relief (these could
even lead to selecting another type of medicine). Medical con-

ditions, other medications you take, and genetic factors should all be considered.

Sometimes patients will hint or ask about trying a particular medicine that was effective for someone they know ("It worked for Ralph!"). Your belief in the effectiveness of that medication could have a powerfully positive influence on that medicine's effectiveness for you via the placebo effect. The placebo effect can also work in a negative direction: if you have heard or believe that a certain antidepressant is bad, then that could have a powerfully negative influence on how it works for you. Despite the importance of the placebo effect and your psychological attitude about a medication, you must consider the factors mentioned in the paragraph above. They are of critical significance and are generally more important in selecting the best medicine for you than what happened to Ralph.

Fortunately, thanks to those unsung heroes who work in the research laboratories whom we never get to meet personally, there are many effective medications available. In the United States, there are over twenty antidepressants to choose from. If drug A does not help, or if troublesome side effects occur with drug A, there is always drug B, or drug C, and so on. Finding the right medicine to treat depression, OCD, or any psychiatric disease is the same as treating high blood pressure, heart disease, or any other physical disease: you keep working with the individual until you find the medicine(s) that works best for that individual.

🌿 Case Example

> Don, the psychiatrist would learn later, had symptoms of obsessive-compulsive disorder dating back to the fourth or fifth grade, but he had always lived with them and had never come to the attention of a mental health professional until this year. Early in the year, he'd experienced a knee injury which required surgery, and he had been unable to work out for the month before his severe symptoms began. He and his therapist later agreed that this change in his

routine may have been the primary stressor that triggered the increase in his symptoms.

It started with the fear that he might come down with AIDS. Many, many years ago, before the AIDS epidemic began sweeping the United States, Don had unprotected sexual relations with a woman who had a history of drug abuse. His "AIDS phobia" stemmed from his thinking that he may have caught the virus from this woman. The "phobia" was actually more of an obsession, for the thoughts about his getting AIDS bombarded his mind every day and he couldn't get rid of them. He also began wondering if he was homosexual, and he couldn't get rid of this thought either. But it was the fear of AIDS that led him to his family doctor to get a blood test. The doctor assured him that he had no signs or symptoms of AIDS and that his "exposure" was at a time that it was extremely unlikely that he could have caught HIV. A blood test for HIV was, sure enough, negative.

During the follow-up visit, his doctor astutely picked up on Don's obsessive fear and delved further into what was going on in Don's mind. Upon hearing Don's history, the doctor referred him to a specialist for psychiatric care. Don had had a very traumatic childhood. His alcoholic father was explosive and had chased Don and his siblings with a butcher knife on more than one occasion. Don remembered the occasion "like it was yesterday" when his drunken father was passed out in bed, and Don was tempted to get the butcher knife and stab him. Don remembered having a "germ phobia" as far back as grade school. He was afraid somebody in his family might catch some "bad germ" and get sick or die. He always washed the silverware and dishes an extra time and made sure the counters were sparkling clean. Throughout his childhood, he frequently washed his hands, especially when he came into the house from outside, and before he touched anything that belonged to another family member. His hands were always red and chafed, and in the winter, they would crack and bleed.

Now, however, his fear was more focused on the AIDS virus and the fact that he might be or become homosexual. He said he felt fearful "99 percent of the time," and he couldn't concentrate because of the constant intrusive thoughts. The psychiatrist began Don on an antipsychotic—a medicine that helps people keep in touch with reality and keep their train of thought—and arranged for Don to see a psychologist for psychotherapy. Despite several dose adjustments while on the antipsychotic tranquilizer, Don did not improve, and he began getting depressed. An antidepressant was added to the tranquilizer, and Don and his psychiatrist worked together on trying to find a dose of each medicine that would give him relief.

About this time, the new generation antidepressants were becoming available, and Don's psychiatrist had had some luck with some other patients who took them. Moreover, preliminary research reports were appearing that showed the effectiveness of these new generation antidepressants in treating OCD symptoms. Don and his doctor agreed to stop his current antidepressant, which had not been doing much, and try a new one. It wasn't a miracle drug, but it helped some. His depressive symptoms improved significantly, and his obsessive thoughts and fears abated by about half, according to his estimate. Don continued in psychotherapy and tried two more of the new generation antidepressants. Side effects occurred at times. Don and his doctor worked well as a team, however, in trying to minimize side effects and maximize benefit. Eventually, Don felt really good. His AIDS phobia and fear of being homosexual disappeared. He continued to be a "clean freak" (as he was fondly referred to by his friends), but he was no longer as driven to wash things so much. Don recovered, but it had taken attempts with five different medicines before the right one was found.

Two Birds with One Stone

Don was lucky in that his medicine actually gave him relief from two disorders: depression and OCD. Because the antidepressants are effective for a variety of psychiatric disorders, this "killing two birds with one stone" can happen with other combinations of symptoms. Consider the case of David.

🌿 Case Example

David had never been a good student. He vividly remembered how his parents would tell him that he had a good brain and then beg him to use it. He rarely studied in junior high or high school but was still able to make good enough grades to go to college. He dropped out of college, however, after a poor performance his freshman year. In high school, he never thought there was anything wrong with him other than he just didn't like to study. But in college, he had really tried. However, he just couldn't seem to concentrate when he tried to study. He would get easily distracted by almost any movement or noise around him, and his mind would wander even when he was able to find an isolated place to study.

After dropping out of college, David held a variety of jobs. He did okay if the job description required good interpersonal skills (such as sales). But his paperwork and reports frequently contained errors, and he was criticized for being disorganized. Eventually, he did find a steady job, and though he did not set the world on fire with his performance, at least he had a job and was able to support himself.

Fortunately, David's social skills were much better than his ability to study. He was gay, had come out of the closet, and was well liked by everybody who met him. However, his love life began to go sour. He had no problem initiating relationships; he was decent-looking and had a great sense of humor. The problem, he was told by his friends, was that he was too "irresponsible" for someone to consider living with him or getting serious with him. As time went by, his want of a long-term relationship grew. He was great fun to be with, but no one seemed interested in making a commitment to him. David had to admit to himself that he was a bit like Oscar in The Odd Couple: *sloppy and disorganized, frequently tardy, and always looking for something he had lost.*

David became mild to moderately depressed, sought professional help for personal improvement, and began seeing a therapist. Around that time, David's sister was having trouble with her ten-year-old son, who was diagnosed as having attention deficit/hyperactivity disorder (ADHD). His sister learned more about ADHD, how it can run in families, and told David she wondered if he might have it. David brought it up with his therapist, who admitted that David could have some of the inattention/distractibility portion of ADHD. Psychological testing was performed and was consistent with an inattention/distractibility problem, and David was referred for a medication evaluation.

David's depression was not striking. In fact, he did not look *depressed to the psychiatrist, but he reported a significant drop in his mood and how much he enjoyed life over the past year. Life was a drag now. Where life used to be fun, and he used to look forward to it (especially the weekends), now it felt as if he was "just putting in time." His energy was down and he slept more than he used to. David said he'd rank the degree of his depression as about a 5 or 6 on a 0–10 scale.*

Similarly, the psychiatrist was not impressed with David's signs and symptoms of ADHD. He had none of the hyperactivity/impulsivity symptoms, and the history of inattention/distractibility problems could also be explained by David's loose, laid-back approach to living in general. Nevertheless, David seemed sincere in describing his pain and his desire for help, so they discussed trying an antidepressant that could, in theory, help with either the depression or the inattention/distractibility or both.

David lucked out. With the first antidepressant they tried, he was feeling better in a month. Not only was his previous good mood back again, now he seemed able to concentrate better. It was most noticeable at work. Now he was able to sit in meetings and focus long enough to grasp the main points of a presentation. Furthermore, where he previously would start one task at work, get up, and begin something else, then flip to another task, he now felt more organized, could prioritize, and could stay on one task longer. David continued working with his therapist and continued on the medication. Two years later David was involved in a long-term relationship that was going well and was getting an A and a B in college courses he was taking in night school.

The co-occurrence of depression and another psychiatric disorder happens fairly frequently. It happens often enough, in fact, that psychiatrists are careful not to miss a coexisting, subtle case of depression in a patient presenting with OCD, panic disorder, alcoholism, PTSD, etc., or to overlook a second diagnosis in a patient presenting with depression.

One Bird with Two Stones

David was lucky, not only to experience relief from two disorders with one medicine but also to have found the "right medicine" on the first try. Often people need to try more than one antidepressant before they find the one that works for them, and sometimes they need a combination of two medicines. Alice was such a person.

✑ CASE EXAMPLE

Alice first entered psychiatric treatment while in her thirties, when she was so depressed that she required hospitalization. Looking back even further than that, Alice remembers times in high school that she would cry "just out of the blue, for no reason." She would stay home from school with physical symptoms which the doctor was unable to explain, sometimes staying in bed for a week. She'd had multiple therapists and psychiatrists over the past thirty years. She said she was "therapied out." She had been on and off multiple antidepressants and had constantly been taking something for the past fifteen years. Despite what sounded like a horrible history, Alice had been able to function at a fairly high level. She had graduated from college, worked outside the home, and been promoted to leadership positions. She had been married for forty years and had raised two daughters, both of whom graduated from college, married and had children, and were successfully working outside the home. Several years ago, however, Alice experienced her worst depression ever. "I was almost catatonic," she said. She was so impaired that she got confused while driving, and her family wondered if she had Alzheimer's disease. A neurological workup, however, was normal.

Alice's psychiatric treatment was stepped up in intensity at that time and she improved, but she never really came "all the way back." She still dreaded being with others and barely left home. It wasn't that she was fearful of leaving home (like an agoraphobic), she just had absolutely no desire to talk or interact with anyone. She was tired all the time and became quite easily fatigued. She was able to do the grocery shopping, which was about all she did outside the home, and she cooked, cleaned, worked around the yard, and "rested." She had been on the same antidepressant at the same dose for over a year and had settled into this lifestyle. A change in her insurance company and Medicare arrangements resulted in her seeing a new psychiatrist.

After she and the new psychiatrist met, they agreed that Alice had experienced a partial *response to the current dose of the antidepressant she was on now. The psychiatrist then challenged her acceptance of this partial response as "the best that can be done." Alice said she had tried a higher dose of her present antidepressant but was unable to tolerate the side effects. She was on one of the new generation antidepressants and said she liked it better than any of the others she had been on before. She handed her new doctor a list of the twelve antidepressants she had tried before. "No thanks," she said. "I'm doing okay. I've been on the others. This works just as well, if not better, and has fewer side effects. I don't want to try anything different."*

Yes, Alice had been on twelve other antidepressants, but she had not yet tried any combination *treatment. Her doctor persuaded her to try adding an old faithful antidepressant (one that she had been on before) to her current new generation antidepressant. Alice tried it and eventually enjoyed a robust response. In three months, she was playing golf weekly, attending church, and having friends over for dinner.*

As researchers discover more and more of the brain's complex chemistry, it comes as no surprise that two antidepressants, working on different parts of the brain, can sometimes be more effective than one. Using two antidepressants, however, is usually tried only in "stubborn" cases that have not responded to conventional treatment with a single antidepressant (monotherapy).

GENERICS AND FORMULARY MEDICINES

Approximately half of the antidepressants in the United States have a generic substitute available. Patients taking antidepressants that have a generic equivalent are invariably curious about taking the generic alternative.

Theoretically, generic medication is supposed to be as good as brand-name medication. Theoretically, they contain the same active chemical ingredient. In reality, though, you never know. In reality, there could be a difference between the brand-name drug and the generic substitute due to the ability or inability of either pharmaceutical company to manufacture a pure product. Are the manufacturing techniques of generic pharmaceutical companies as good as the manufacturing techniques of the brand-name pharmaceutical companies? Sweeping stereotypes about generics in general don't always apply, for there are a variety of companies that manufacture generic medication, and all generics are not the same. It would be nice to have scientifically controlled experiments that compare the effectiveness of each brand-name drug with its generic substitute, but such studies do not exist.

The purity and quality of *your* antidepressant is the issue for you, so if you are considering taking a generic substitute, forget sweeping stereotypes about generics. Just worry about the medicine you are taking. Ask your physician; he or she may have some experience with or knowledge about the generic substitute of your particular medicine.

Formulary medicines are those medications that your insurance company or your managed-care organization prefers that you take. Be it for high blood pressure, acid stomach, depression, or whatever, the health insurance industry and managed-care industry often separate the medicines available for a given condition into formulary and nonformulary medicines. The medicines on their formulary list are judged to be at least as good as the nonformulary medicines, but more cost-effective. These lists are distributed to the doctors treating the patients who are enrolled in these programs.

Insurance companies and managed-care organizations offer financial incentives to steer their enrollees toward using formulary and generic medication. Of course they do, because it saves them money! They do this by lowering their reimbursement rate (i.e., the patient pays more out-of-pocket) for nonformulary and brand-name medicines.

At times there are valid medical reasons to use a nonformulary medicine. For example, the patient may not have responded to a formulary medicine but did respond to a nonformulary medicine. When this is true, a reasonable insurance company or managed-care organization will not penalize the patient for using the nonformulary medicine. In such cases, however, the fiscal intermediary will require proof and documentation that there is a valid medical necessity to use the nonformulary medicine. Providing this documentation is inconvenient for the patient (and the doctor), but it does result in significant cost savings for the patient.

21

Finding the Right Dose

JUST AS THERE IS NO one antidepressant medication that works for everybody, there is no one dose that works for everybody. Again, everyone is different. Effective treatment requires finding the right dose of the right medicine for each individual, and finding that dose requires the teamwork and patience of the "therapeutic alliance" discussed earlier.

The *total daily dose* of the medicine (the amount ingested every twenty-four hours) is what doctors focus on when trying to find the right dose. Whether to take this dose all at once or to divide it up, and *when* to take it, are questions we will address in the next chapter.

Medical research has established what is generally the starting "target" dose for each antidepressant. However, other factors must be considered before selecting the starting dose for each individual: factors such as other medical conditions, other medications being taken, previous experience with antidepressants, body characteristics, and the patient's age. For a variety of physiological reasons, as people get older, they usually respond at a lower dose than what is required at a younger age.

Sometimes, at the start, a dose is selected that is intentionally lower than the target dose. This dose is then gradually ratcheted upward every few days or every week until the actual target dose is reached. Other times, people start immediately at the target dose on the first day. It all depends on which antidepressant is being used and the individual using it.

Once the patient reaches the target dose (what is hoped to be the therapeutic dose), physicians usually recommend a three-to-four-week waiting period (see Chapter 19, "Aesop's Tortoise") to see if this dose will work as hoped. The length of the waiting period varies with the individual, however. A variety of factors may shorten it or lengthen it. For example, when treating a patient who is *severely* depressed or in a hospital, the doctor may recommend not waiting the entire three to four weeks. In such a case, a more aggressive approach would be to nudge the dose up another notch every week or two, or even faster. On the other hand, a patient may become medically ill or may have some unexplained physical symptoms (which could be side effects) during the three-to-four-week waiting period. The patient may have a particularly stressful personal life during this three- or four-week wait, making it difficult to accurately assess the response to the drug. Or maybe a patient is just beginning to show some improvement at week three or four. In such cases, the physician may recommend waiting a couple of more weeks before changing anything. The general rule is to wait three or four weeks at what is hoped will be the therapeutic dose, and see what happens. To achieve a robust response with minimal side effects at this initial target dose is, of course, wonderful. It also makes the next step easy: don't change anything. Keep it the same. "If it ain't broke, don't fix it."

What happens if there is only minimal or no improvement at the end of the waiting period? A change is made. Usually, the physician recommends that the dose of the medicine be increased. Sometimes the dose may even be decreased. Sometimes another medication may be added to boost or "augment" the first medicine. Sometimes the current medication is discontinued and a switch is made to another medicine. In any event, time is critical. No matter what change is made, it takes more time for the new regimen to kick in. If that does not work, the dose or the medicine must be changed once more. And again, you need to wait.

If intolerable side effects occur at any point, the same rule applies: the dose and/or the medicine are changed. And again, you must wait. As you can see, the general operating principle is (1) to give a selected dose enough time for improvement to occur, and (2) if insufficient improvement or intolerable side effects occur, change the dose or change the medicine, then (3) give the new regimen enough time for improvement to occur.

Never adjust your own dose unilaterally, without any discussion with your doctor (see Chapter 27, "Unilateral Dose Adjustments"). Finding the right dose of the right medicine is the job of the team—not you alone.

Case Example

Diane got caught shoplifting—again. It was about the tenth time she had been caught. The arresting officer even knew her. He had been to court for her trial on a previous occasion and knew she wasn't your ordinary thief. Diane's record listed what she had been caught stealing before, but it was not the profile of a thief stealing for her own gain. Her court record had her labeled as a kleptomaniac, and the judge had previously ordered her to seek professional help. Diane saw a therapist for about one year but said it did no good. When the impulse to steal got too strong, she just couldn't resist it. On one occasion she had to spend the weekend in jail, but even the thought of having to repeat that experience was not strong enough to resist the kleptomaniac impulse.

The policeman liked Diane and felt sorry for her. He spoke to her like a fond uncle. "Why don't you tell your doctor about it and see if he can help?" Diane had a good relationship with her ob/gyn, who had delivered her baby. Ashamed as she was, she swallowed her pride and told her doctor, who started her on one of the new genera-

tion antidepressants and referred her to a psychiatrist. Diane admit-ted she'd had this problem since she was about twelve years old and guessed she had stolen an average of twenty-five to fifty items per year ever since. It was more likely to happen when she was depressed or tense, or "hyped-up." Two of her relatives had been institutional-ized, though she knew of no other kleptomania in the family.

Diane began in psychotherapy again. Her therapist advised her never to go into a store or other place where she might steal unless she was accompanied by a "buddy" who knew about her problem. Di-ane had a large family, and with all her arrests, her problem was no secret. Several of her siblings said they would be happy to help her out and to act as her "buddy." The antidepressants seemed to calm and relax Diane at first, but that effect wore off after about two weeks. In five weeks, the anxiety and tension had returned. Diane recognized the hyped-up feeling, and the impulse to steal began poking her again.

Thinking maybe she was on too much medicine, her psychiatrist lowered the dose. He reasoned that, since she felt better early on (before the medicine had the entire three to four weeks of cumulative activity), maybe Diane was someone who needed a dose lower than the conventional starting dose. They waited three weeks, but this did not work. They then agreed to increase the dose to double what Diane had started out on, wait a month, and see what happened. Of course, all this time, Diane continued to see her therapist weekly.

One month later Diane reported she was feeling good again. Interestingly, though she had initially denied any sleep problem, she now said that she was sleeping wonderfully. The tense, depressed, hyped-up feeling had only flared up on her a few times in the past week. And Diane had now gone weeks without stealing anything— the longest she'd gone since she was twelve years old.

22

Know When to Take It

THE ANTIDEPRESSANTS WORK via the cumulative, ongoing activity in the brain, and this transformation takes several weeks (see Chapter 19, "Aesop's Tortoise"). Theoretically, then, it should not matter what time of day you take your medicine. Theoretically, what should matter is that you get the entire dose into your body every day so that it can perform its daily activity. It is this *long-term* effect that you are after.

For the most part, this theory is true, but there are some exceptions. Some antidepressants need to be taken at intervals throughout the day (two, three, or even four times a day) or at a certain time in relation to eating food. Spreading the total daily dose into these "divided doses" optimizes the benefits of these particular drugs and helps prevent side effects. However, for most antidepressants, it usually does not matter if the total day's dose is spread out or taken all at once. You should do whatever works best for you. Ask your physician if your dose needs to be spread out, or timed with food, or if it is optional.

Let's examine how the option of taking it whenever you

desire can get rid of unwanted side effects that occasionally occur. Even though it is the *long-term* effect that you are after, you may feel a *short-term* effect one-half hour or several hours after you take a dose. This short-term effect may be experienced as something negative (e.g., the medicine may make you feel too sleepy during the day). With the option of taking it whenever you desire, you merely take the dose late in the evening. The "side effect" of sleepiness then occurs when it is time for bed, which may actually help you get a good night's sleep, and then wears off by morning.

🌿 CASE EXAMPLE

Katherine's headaches were making life miserable for her. All her life she'd had maybe a few more headaches than the average person, but never any like these. These were severe *headaches, and they didn't get any better with over-the-counter medications. She went to her internist, wondering if these were migraines. No, they weren't migraines, she found out. Her doctor called them muscle-contraction/ tension headaches. Stronger pain medicine was prescribed, and it helped, but the headaches kept coming back. Katherine returned to her doctor, who suggested she try an antidepressant.*

Katherine had taken an antidepressant several years earlier. She'd had aches and pains in her bones and joints, felt stiff (particularly in the mornings), and had been so tired that she wondered if she had chronic fatigue syndrome. Her doctor had diagnosed fibromyalgia (a syndrome involving muscle stiffness and pain) and prescribed, among other things, an antidepressant. However, the antidepressant made her so sleepy that she discontinued it. The fibromyalgia symptoms had never gone completely away, though they had improved with other medication. Many women her age seemed to have similar aches and stiffness, so Katherine figured she would just live with it.

Other than these symptoms and a mild problem with her weight, Katherine was in good health. She didn't think she was depressed and she asked her internist why she wanted to put her on an an-

tidepressant. The doctor explained simply that the antidepressants often help with headaches. "There are theories about why, just like there are theories about why it helps fibromyalgia," she said. "I don't know if the theories are true or not. All I know is that quite a few of my patients experience pain relief from the antidepressants." Katherine agreed to try one, as long as it wasn't the same one that had made her so sleepy a few years ago. Her instructions were to take one-half tablet twice per day.

Unfortunately, Katherine became sleepy on this dosage. She could barely stay awake after lunch, so she called her doctor. "Stop the morning dose. Just take the one-half tablet at night only for five nights, then take a full tablet at night until your next appointment," her doctor advised. Katherine did this, and the sleepiness was gone by her next appointment. She stayed on this dose, and a month later her headaches had almost disappeared entirely. Additionally, she was having fewer aches and pains.

Similarly, the flexibility to take the medicine at any time of day can be advantageous if an antidepressant taken in the evening makes you feel too stimulated or seems to worsen your sleep. Merely take it in the morning. The "side effect" is thereby turned into something positive: an invigorating jump start on your day which wears off by evening.

If an antidepressant makes you feel queasy, take it with food. And any short-term effect can be minimized by dividing the daily dose into several smaller doses, then spreading them out throughout the day. This enables you to still get the required total daily dose, but it will not hit you all at once. Getting a green light to experiment with the time of administration has helped many a patient to conquer problems with side effects.

Most patients, fortunately, will not feel such short-term effects. For most patients, the biggest problem is just plain remembering to take their medicine. Taking it all at once, just once a day, is more convenient and much easier to remember than spreading it out. To prevent forgetting their medicine, patients frequently take it at the same time every day and link it with a routine activity in order to "get into a habit." For example, they may take it in the morning when they brush their teeth or eat breakfast. Some take it later in the day, when they eat their main meal. Others get in the habit of taking it right before they go to bed at night.

Occasionally, it will happen that the most effective dose is to alternate the number of milligrams ingested every other day—for example, taking one capsule one day and two capsules the next day. This may work fine as long as patients remember which day they are supposed to take one and which day they are supposed to take two. A helpful memory device in this situation is for patients to take the odd number of capsules on the odd days of the month and the even number of capsules on the even days of the month.

Most pharmacies sell long, rectangular, plastic boxes (about the size of a harmonica) that have seven compartments: one for each day of the week. This medicine dispenser can be filled every Sunday with your week's supply of medicine and then kept in a location where you will remember it every day at "medicine time." Develop whatever habit helps you to remember to take your total daily dose every day.

At the risk of sounding like a broken record, it still needs mentioning: the most important thing is to *take the total daily dose every day.* Is it okay for you to experiment with *when* you take this total dose? Ask your doctor what he or she recommends for you and the particular medicine you are taking.

What About When I Forget to Take My Antidepressant?

Even the best medicine-takers in the world will occasionally forget to take a dose, or skip a dose for some reason. What should you do when that happens?

Ask your doctor, when the prescription for your antidepressant is first written, what to do if you skip a dose. Most of the time, he or she will say it's okay to go ahead and take your "skipped" dose later that same day. Remember, getting the total daily dose into you every day is what counts. Occasionally, though, your doctor will tell you not to "catch up" later that day (especially with Wellbutrin, which is almost always taken in divided doses).

For all antidepressants, do not try to catch up with a skipped dose by taking it the *next* day. Once your day ends (which is midnight for most people), forget about catching up and just start out again as usual the next morning.

23

Blood Levels

MEASURING THE CONCENTRATION of an antidepressant in the blood of a patient is sometimes helpful, though it depends on which antidepressant you are taking. With a few of the old faithful antidepressants (Pamelor and Norpramin in particular), there is some correlation between their concentration in the blood and their therapeutic effectiveness.

Blood level measurement can be of great value for patients who take one of those few antidepressants. Blood level tests can remove some of the guesswork and experimentation by trial and error when trying to find the right dose of a medicine. For example, if a patient is not responding to a certain dose, and a blood test indicates not enough or too much medicine in the blood, the dosage is merely adjusted up or down accordingly. If the blood test indicates a "therapeutic concentration" of the medicine in the blood, but the patient is not improving, then that medicine is probably not the correct medicine for that patient. A switch to another drug is then made.

If you have the antidepressant level measured in your blood, it is important to remember several things: (1) When research defines a "therapeutic blood level" of an antidepressant, this definition is based on what is therapeutic for most people, *not everybody*. These numbers are not hard-and-fast; there are exceptions. Some patients do best on blood levels that are lower or higher than what is the alleged "therapeutic range." (2) As one of my wise old professors once told me, "You treat the patient, not the laboratory test." How the patient is doing is what is important. The blood test is merely an aid to help the patient get better. (3) Blood tests are not done routinely. They are primarily used when a patient is not making progress. (4) The measurement will not be meaningful until the *same* total daily dose of the medicine has been taken for enough days in a row to reach a steady, stable equilibrium in the blood. This usually takes a week or two. (5) The timing of when the blood gets drawn is crucial. Usually, to be meaningful, it must be drawn between ten and twelve hours after the last dose.

If you are not progressing on schedule, ask your doctor about the possibility of measuring the blood level of the antidepressant you are taking.

⚘ Case Example

Mary had been diagnosed with depression a year earlier and had been doing everything her doctors told her to do. She had been seeing her psychologist every week and, in fact, had learned a great deal from her therapy. She started walking at least four times a week and now found that it was not quite the drudgery it had been when she first started walking. She took a vitamin daily and was eating more nutritiously than she had in years. Mary was better, but there was still a lot of room for improvement, and her family doctor referred her to a psychiatrist.

After a few false starts with some antidepressants that had no effect on Mary, the psychiatrist prescribed one of the old faithful antidepressants. When Mary didn't respond to it, the doctor increased the dose, and Mary's pharmacist commented that it struck him as rather high. Mary looked it up in a drug book and learned

she was on the maximum recommended dose. Fortunately, this an-
tidepressant was one whose clinical effectiveness was known to corre-
late with blood levels. The psychiatrist recommended that Mary have
her blood drawn "to see how much of the medicine that you're
taking is actually getting into your blood." Mary went along with it,
though she wondered what good it would do since she was already on
the highest maximum dose.

When Mary was told that the blood level report indicated that the
concentration of the antidepressant was well below the therapeutic
range, she was puzzled. "I swear I'm taking it every day, Doctor; I
can't understand this. It's the brand drug; I'm not taking a ge-
neric." Mary's doctor explained, "It's not your fault. You are just a
fast metabolizer." "A fast what? *What's that?"*

The doctor explained that different people's bodies metabolize or
break down medications at different rates. "It's like some people are
very short and some are very tall, but most people are somewhere in
the middle. Some people break these drugs down quickly and urinate
them out quickly. Others are the opposite and break these drugs
down slowly and urinate them out slowly, but most people are in the
middle. You, however, happen to be in group number one: a fast
metabolizer."

"But I don't urinate that much," Mary said. The doctor went
on, "Actually, it doesn't have anything to do with how much *you*
urinate. It has to do with your liver just eating up this drug like Pac-
Man. You excrete it in your normal urine volume, so you don't even
know it is happening."

Cautiously, they raised Mary's dose another notch and checked
another blood level. It was still low. However, one "raise" later and
one month later, Mary felt like she was over the hump. She was
amazed. She was taking well over the dosage that her book had said
was the maximum, ceiling dose, and she barely had any side ef-
fects—just some mild dry mouth. "It's not how much you take by
mouth that matters," her psychiatrist reiterated. "It's how much
you get into your blood, and from your blood, into your brain."

24

Peaks and Valleys,
Chunks of Time

THE ROAD TO RECOVERY is not straight. Expect peaks and valleys on your road to recovery. Nobody's symptoms stay the same for long periods of time; symptoms fluctuate in their frequency and severity. Everybody has a bad day, or a few bad days in a row, from time to time. This is true whether one is recovering from depression, obsessive-compulsive disorder, bulimia, or whatever. So, do not let a "valley" fool you into thinking you are doing worse than you really are. *Patients not forewarned about this will, when they hit those inevitable valleys, think that the psychotherapy and/or the medication is not working.* This lack of hope and faith in the treatment can then undermine the determination and positive attitude that help fuel the fight against the illness. This negativism can begin a self-fulfilling prophecy that leads to treatment failure. *Do not let this happen to you.*

These peaks and valleys make it difficult to evaluate whether progress is being made. If you measure your progress by picking one point in time, and that point happens to be in a valley, you may be misled into thinking that you are not making progress. If you pick a point in time that happens to be on a peak, you may be misled into thinking that you are doing better than you really are. If you pick several different points in time, some of which are in valleys and some of which are on peaks, you will not know whether you are getting worse or getting better. You will feel like patients who say, "I'm all over the map, Doc; I don't know whether I'm coming or going."

In order to accurately evaluate whether or not progress is being made, you and your doctor must take a *chunk* of time and look at how the symptoms have *averaged* over that chunk of time. Remember, though, that this chunk of time must be long enough to get a true average. If it is too short, a series of peaks for several days in a row can artificially raise the average. Similarly, a series of valleys for several days in a row can artificially take the average down. The chunk of time must be of sufficient length to account for such sustained fluctuations. Generally, a week or two is a big enough chunk. Then take a similar-sized chunk of time from several weeks or a month ago. Look at the symptoms' average back then and compare the two averages.

🌿 CASE EXAMPLE

Ruth went through one of the most horrible freak-accident experiences her psychiatrist could imagine. It was one of those that you pray to God will never happen to you or your family and that, when you hear about it, immediately makes you stop feeling sorry for yourself over small things. Ruth's daughter and grandchildren were visiting her on a beautiful Easter afternoon. It was balmy and the children went outside to play. They loved to run and roll down the long hill in the front yard, which they had done hundreds of times before. The children were well trained not to leave the yard and knew ''┘y'd better never, ever go into the* *street. Consequently, the adults didn't feel obligated to keep an eye on the kids.*

Ruth was in the kitchen when she heard the scream. She ran outside and saw her car at the bottom of the hill. The car had been parked in front of the garage at the top of the hill, but Ruth's youngest granddaughter had climbed into the driver's seat and taken the gearshift lever out of Park. Apparently, it had rolled backward down the hill, and in doing so, it had run over her little grandson, including his head. Ruth was the first to the body, and she knew right away there was nothing that could be done. She even saw what she thought looked like brain on the asphalt.

This terrible accident occurred several months before Ruth ever made it to the psychiatrist's office. She'd been "heavily sedated" by her family physician and was able to make it through the funeral. She remained on the sedatives and tranquilizers but essentially hadn't been able to function, let alone return to work. Ruth barely slept and had huge, dark half-circles under her eyes. She was afraid to go to sleep and she fought sleep because of the nightmares. The nightmares were "just like being back there again when it happened." During the day, she seemed as if she was in a trance half the time, and she'd occasionally jump with fright when someone tried to get her attention. Sometimes, when she was in the kitchen, she thought she could hear a scream. She was pelted with flashbacks of the scene every day and couldn't get the image of her grandson's body and smashed head out of her mind's eye. She could still see the brain matter on the asphalt. Ruth had no appetite, barely ate, and lost twenty-five pounds.

Ruth was started in intensive psychotherapy and on antidepressant medication. Warned about the "lag time" before the antidepressant would "kick in," Ruth willingly took it every day. However, after a month of trying, she declared, "Okay, I've given it time to kick in, but it's not doing a thing. I only slept about two hours last night, and I'm still having nightmares and flashbacks. Let's get off this stuff." Not willing to give up so easily, her doctor asked Ruth to compare how bad the nightmares, *flashbacks, and insomnia had been over the past week with how bad they had been in the week prior to starting the medicine. Ruth reflected, then admitted they hadn't been quite as bad. Her dose was increased and her psychiatrist encouraged her to continue taking it religiously, and to not judge her progress by how she was doing at any one point in time. "Take a chunk of time and compare averages," she advised.*

A month later Ruth knew she was better. Yes, she still had trouble believing that the accident had really happened; she still felt stunned and numb, but she felt more "with it" than she had six weeks ago, and quite a few others had commented to her that she didn't look like such a zombie. She wasn't sleeping well, but at least the nightmares were coming less frequently, and she wasn't afraid of going to sleep anymore. She was getting four to five hours of sleep per night now. "I'm up and down, Doctor. Some days the flashbacks are terrible, and some nights I hardly sleep at all, but overall I'm better. My appetite is gone, but at least I can stomach food part of the time, and I haven't lost any more weight." Also, very importantly, her ability to think and comprehend was periodically showing up again. Her participation in group therapy varied from day to day, but at times she was able to converse and pay attention to others in the group.

Ruth's ability to benefit from therapy vacillated from day to day, but slowly improved. It took an entire year before Ruth was able to return to work. A year later, when reflecting with her therapist about her progress, she said, "I'll never get over what happened, but at least I'm back amongst the living again."

Nobody gets well overnight. As we discussed in Chapter 19, the antidepressants take three or four weeks (or longer) to kick in, and improvement is slow. They kick in so gradually and subtly that improvement is not noticeable from one day to the next. This tortoiselike movement also makes it difficult to evaluate whether or not progress is being made. Comparing your current weekly average with your average of a month ago is a good measure of your actual progress. What you are looking for is a *trend* toward improvement. If there has been no trend, or if there was previously a positive trend but it has now leveled off and you are on a plateau, a change needs to be made. If comparing your averages indicates a trend in the right direction, then stay on course.

25

When and If to
Stop an Antidepressant

ONCE PATIENTS FINALLY ACHIEVE satisfactory symptom relief (if not before), they begin to wonder how long they should stay on their medication. Some patients, particularly those who had some reluctance to taking medicine in the first place or who are frightened of being dependent on a medication, want to get off their medicine as soon as possible. Others, fearful of backsliding without the medication, would just as soon stay on it indefinitely. How do you know what is the best thing to do?

Depression

CONTINUATION THERAPY

During the 1950s and 1960s, there were no guidelines about when to discontinue medicine when treating depression. Patients and doctors more or less winged it. Since then, beautifully designed research has made it absolutely clear what should be done for people recovering from their first episode of depression: stay on the medication for at least six months of stability before discontinuation. The clock measuring the six months starts ticking when the patient's symptoms have disappeared, not when the medication was started.

Researchers have discovered that the first six months or so after a patient's symptoms disappear is a period of very high risk for a return of the symptoms. In fact, the term "recovery" is not used until a patient has been symptom-free for about a year. The wonderful news is that staying on an antidepressant during this risk period *significantly* lowers the risk of having a relapse. Continuing on the medication for the next six months after your symptoms disappear is referred to as "continuation therapy."

Researchers have also discovered, however, that some people (a much smaller percent) who religiously take their medicine every day will still have a return of their symptoms. Staying on the medicine, then, is no *guarantee* that the symptoms will not return. However, the data clearly showed that the statistical odds of relapse are *much* lower if the antidepressant is continued. If you like playing the odds, stay on the medicine for at least the next six months.

CASE EXAMPLE

Dawn was stunningly beautiful. She had almond-shaped, green eyes over high cheekbones and thick, dark hair. She was so pretty and young-looking that her psychiatrist could not believe she was the mother of six children. "I'm so lucky," she later told him. "Lucky to have lived through my twenties, let alone have six children that I love dearly."

Around twenty years earlier and weighing less than ninety pounds, Dawn had gone into a coma and almost died from an electrolyte imbalance. Her illness back then was diagnosed as "dehydration, stomach flu, and stress." She received counseling for the stress and was able to talk to her therapist about her personal life and all the "stress" without revealing that her weight loss was actually self-induced. Back then, anorexia nervosa had even more of a stigma than it has now, and Dawn did not tell anyone her secret. The counseling helped, and Dawn controlled her anorexic behaviors enough that she survived and, in fact, married soon thereafter.

Thin was in and Dawn was gorgeous, so she'd had many suitors. She married a handsome and intelligent young man who became financially successful while Dawn was having babies. Over the years, Dawn was continually bombarded by other women in the community with complimentary remarks like "How do you keep so thin?" On the one hand, Dawn enjoyed the attention and the compliments. On the other hand, she was in a secret hell. Every day was a struggle— an internal battle of will to stick to her strict, self-induced diet. More and more her willpower alone was not sufficient, and she began to depend on diet pills and laxatives for help. Occasionally, she'd lose control and go into a feeding frenzy, then make herself vomit what she ate. That didn't happen very often, though, because she hated to vomit.

Dawn grew to hate her illness (over the years, as more information about anorexia nervosa became public, she'd learned that it was an illness). She realized she was obsessed with her weight, but she couldn't stop herself from thinking about it or force herself to change her habitual behaviors. She loved her children more than life itself, but her thoughts about food kept intruding into her consciousness, and in her heart she knew she wasn't focusing on her children and their activities as much as a mother should. The children often seemed to be a bother. Eventually, it wore her down, and over the next year Dawn got depressed. She continued to be obsessed with her diet and her weight, but new thoughts began creeping in. Dawn would be washing the dishes, reading the paper, or doing practically anything, and she would catch herself staring off into nowhere, thinking thoughts of how bad a mother she was and that she was essentially a worthless person. A feeling of emptiness grew inside her. She felt like crying and, in fact, wished she could cry—but nothing came out.

Dawn didn't want to talk to anybody or do anything—she just wanted to be left alone. She gradually began spending more time alone. When she was with her children, she would snap at them for little things. Seconds later she would tell herself, "Come on, now, they're just being children," and then feel more worthless and guilty for being "such a bitch." She was even more hostile to her husband, who soon told her she'd better get her act together or he was out of there. Dawn had never really been very sexually inclined to begin with, and her interest in sex fell from low to zero. Before, she'd at least occasionally have sex in order to please her husband; now she wasn't even doing that. Of course, this didn't do much for her marriage.

Things went from bad to worse: Dawn began waking up in the middle of the night or early in the morning. She wondered about just "taking off somewhere," though she didn't know where she would go or what she would do. She wondered about killing herself. Finally, she saw a psychiatrist, and this time she "came clean" about her eating disorder. She was begun on an antidepressant and began seeing the psychiatrist in individual psychotherapy. Additionally, Dawn was referred to a nearby intensive psychotherapy program that specialized in treating eating disorders.

Dawn was highly motivated and did well. Her husband attended the evening family sessions offered by the eating disorders program and proved to be a sensitive and understanding man. Within four months, not only was Dawn out of her depression, she also had a much better handle on her eating disorder. Grateful and confident, one day Dawn thanked her psychiatrist for all his help and said she was ready to go off the medicine now. The psychiatrist reiterated what he'd told her several months earlier, that she should stay on the antidepressant for a period of time—at least six months—and stabilize before going off it. Dawn politely declined. "I'm a new person, Doctor. I know I'm okay—I don't need to be supermodel-thin to be okay. I learned so much from you and the program. I want to do it on my own now; I'm ready."

The psychiatrist could see her point. Dawn had learned a lot, and she was using what she'd learned. He truly believed that much of her improvement was due to the psychotherapy and not just the medicine. Still, he knew the odds: the deck was stacked against her if she discontinued the medicine now. They spent the entire session "discussing" (or arguing) the issue. At the end of the session, they agreed to disagree—the doctor again advising her not to stop the medication but acknowledging that it was her life and her choice to make.

Dawn chose to stop her medicine, which she did. Three months later she was back. "You were right," she said. "Within a month it was back. I tried to fight it for a few weeks, but I couldn't. My husband could tell something was wrong and was pretty upset with me when I told him I had stopped the antidepressant. I finally gave up and went back on it. I could tell the difference in two weeks."

There are no scientifically proven facts explaining why this continuation therapy seems to work. Maybe it gives the brain's chemicals time to stabilize. Maybe it helps give the newly learned information and emotional healing from psychotherapy a chance to sink in. Maybe it gives the patient an opportunity to practice new behaviors, and time for the new behaviors to become second nature. Maybe it simply gives time for the patient's life in general to settle down and get into a more normal routine. Whatever the reasons, a period of continuation therapy works and is a good practice to follow.

IN TIMES OF STRESS

When the continuation therapy phase is up, what then? Just stop it automatically? No. Even after plenty of time for stabilization has passed, medication should not be lowered during times of change or if current stress levels are higher than usual. Similarly, if major changes are *expected in the near future,* or if stress levels are *expected to rise* in the near future, it is not a good time to lower the dose.

Stress, it should be pointed out, can present itself in a wide variety of ways. What for one person may be an "exciting challenge" may be perceived as "stressful" to somebody else. The exact nature of the stressor doesn't matter much. How it is experienced by the patient matters a great deal. A significant change in one's life (e.g., a different job, a new baby, a move) may not be perceived as stressful and may very well be a positive thing. But it is still not a good time to lower the dose. If a relapse were to occur after lowering the dose, you could legitimately ask, "Is the relapse due to everything that is going on right now or due to the reduction in dosage?"

It should also be pointed out that the perfect time to lower a dose is when there is no stress whatsoever, but this is quite a rarity in life. Everybody has at least some stress in his or her life the vast majority of the time. Therefore, it would be impractical to wait to lower the dose until this happens (you could be waiting forever!).

Using the concepts of "usual" and "higher than usual" levels of stress can help guide you and your doctor when it is time to decide whether or not to lower the dose. There is some risk of relapse when the dose is lowered, so it would be foolish to take this risk when you are more vulnerable due to higher-than-usual levels of stress. A guiding principle is to wait until the continuation phase is over, ensure that your stress level is neither higher than usual nor expected to be higher than usual in the near future, then proceed (see Chapter 26, "How to Stop an Antidepressant").

Discontinuing psychotherapy and medication at the same time can cause problems. First of all, yanking both components of treatment away from you all at once may be the equivalent of pulling the rug out from under you: too much, too fast. Secondly, if you do relapse, you do not know if it was the withdrawal from the medicine or the withdrawal from the psychotherapy that caused the problem. Therefore, in order to treat the relapse, both treatment modalities need to be started up again. It is better to first taper off one, then the other, rather than risk a relapse by abruptly withdrawing them both simultaneously.

MAINTENANCE MEDICATION

Research on depression has revealed another vitally important point: some people need to stay on their antidepressant for years. In fact, some people need to stay on it indefinitely to prevent further episodes.

Depression, OCD, panic disorder, and other disorders are, for many, diseases that recur. Staying on medication to prevent further episodes is called maintenance medication. It is similar to how people with asthma take daily medication to prevent further asthma attacks. So, for some, it is not an issue of knowing *when* to stop the medication; the issue is knowing to *never* stop the medication. Be sure to discuss this extremely important issue with your doctor (more about this in Chapter 36, "Relapses and Recurrences").

🌿 Case Example

Ever since junior high school, Melanie had been moodier than her older sister, who was "Miss Everything" at school (popular, excellent grades, cheerleader, class officer, prom queen nominee, and so on). Melanie was especially moody before her menstrual period, and this became sort of a joke in the family and, later on, with her girlfriends too. Mainly, she would get sulky and irritable. She would always come out of it okay, and she never became clinically depressed—until now.

Fortunately, Melanie worked in the medical field and knew about depression and its warning signs, so she recognized it and sought treatment. At first, she didn't want to take any medicine. She had some personal issues she needed to work on, and she and her psychologist appropriately delved into these. But her sleep, in particular, was so disrupted that her psychologist persuaded her to see a physician for possible medication. Melanie responded well to the combination of psychotherapy and antidepressant medication and eventually felt good and slept well again.

During the six-month continuation phase of the antidepressant, Melanie remained stable. In fact, she noticed she had been less moody than she used to be before she ever got depressed, and her PMS had definitely lightened up. Melanie and her psychiatrist mused over whether this was because she was on the antidepressant or because of her psychotherapy (which had been extremely helpful to her). At any rate, they agreed that she should not stay on the antidepressant forever and that since she was going off it someday, now was as good a time as ever.

The continuation phase was over, so they cut the dose back and tapered off the medicine. Within two weeks after her last dose, Melanie was weepy and having difficulty in sleeping again. She tried to "gut it out" and give her body a chance to get used to being off the medicine. "Besides," she thought to herself, "maybe it's just psychological." But it didn't get better, and Melanie did not want to take any chances. She went back on the antidepressant, and within three weeks she was fine again.

Melanie continued taking the antidepressant over the next year. The year went relatively well, and, like before, she thought she'd felt better (including around her menstrual period) on the medicine compared to how she felt before she ever took it. "Maybe it's psychological," she said to her psychiatrist. "Maybe it's that placebo effect thing. But I really don't think I want to be dependent on a medicine. I know I don't want to take it the rest of my life." More than a year passed. Melanie had done well, and there was minimal stress in her life. They agreed to try stopping the medicine again, only this time they went slower—much slower—and Melanie did fine.

Three years later, however, Melanie was back having the same symptoms of depression she'd had before. Also like before, Melanie kept comparing herself to others and kept thinking thoughts like "I'm as good as she is" or "I'm better than her when it comes to . . . ," as if she was trying to defend herself or convince somebody that she was okay. "I'm all hung up on my sister again too," she said, recognizing the pattern. Melanie started psychotherapy again and went back on the same antidepressant that had helped before. Again, she recovered nicely.

This time Melanie stayed in psychotherapy for a year. They worked on her self-esteem, her competition with her sister, the effect that her feelings about her sister had on her relationship with others, and so on, until they both agreed they could only beat a dead horse so long. They also discussed her parents and her childhood and, of course, her current life situation. Both Melanie and her psychologist felt she was really a pretty balanced and mentally healthy woman. Meanwhile, Melanie had stayed on her antidepressant.

Six months after Melanie and her psychologist terminated psychotherapy, Melanie was ready once again to try to go off her medicine. Like before, they went very slowly. Months went by, and things went well until Melanie was almost off her medicine. In fact, she was taking the smallest-sized dose manufactured, and was only taking it every other day, when the insomnia began again. They bumped the dose back up to once daily, and Melanie slept okay. A few months later they tried going to every other day again. But again, Melanie became sad, tired, and slept poorly.

That was enough for Melanie and her doctor. That was eleven years ago. Ever since then, Melanie has taken one dose every morning with her fruit juice. She has had no further episodes of depression and she swears she's been happier than she had ever been before (and her PMS is gone).

Other Disorders

There are no hard-and-fast, scientifically proven guidelines on when to stop the antidepressants when treating OCD, panic disorder, generalized anxiety disorder, social phobia, the eating disorders, PTSD, ADHD, OCD-related disorders, and other disorders. However, the unwritten rule that most doctors follow is to recommend a period of continuation medication, just as if they were treating depression. In fact, patients with panic disorder do better if their continuation therapy goes on for a year or more. After the continuation therapy phase is completed, the antidepressant may then be weaned, depending on the individual and the diagnosis.

As a rule, out of all patients with disorders other than depression, the ones most likely to do well after stopping an antidepressant are those whose symptoms are of recent onset. Disorders like ADHD and premenstrual dysphoric disorder are ongoing and persistent, and therefore require maintenance medication. Unfortunately, it is not uncommon for any of these other disorders to become ongoing and persistent, and therefore require maintenance medication. All over the world, doctors who have used these medicines for years agree that some people with these disorders need maintenance medicine indefinitely, just as some people with depression need maintenance medicine indefinitely.

26

How to Stop an Antidepressant

WHEN IT IS TIME TO STOP the antidepressant, how do you do it? Just stop it abruptly? It depends. If the daily dosage is already quite low, there may be no need to even consider a slow wean off the drug, and the answer is "Yes, just stop it abruptly." But, in most cases, it makes sense to slowly taper off the medicine in a controlled, step-wise fashion. This gives the brain time to adjust to "taking over on its own" without the help of the medicine.

Furthermore, this slow taper gives the patient and the doctor an opportunity to see what happens at each level as the dosage is stepped down. Should relapse occur at any one of the lower levels, the dose is usually raised back up again. But it may not be necessary to raise the dose all the way back to where you started from. However, if the dose *is* raised all the way back to where you started from, you may not have to keep it there long. With the experience of successfully tapering down, step by step, before the relapse occurred, you have "documented proof" of doing well at lower doses. You may do fine just keeping the dose at one of these lower levels for a while before trying again to taper completely off. Or if you end up on long-term maintenance medication, you have a track record of effectiveness at the "lowest possible dose."

Additionally, some of the antidepressants can cause a "discontinuation syndrome" (withdrawal symptoms) in certain people if they are abruptly stopped (also see Chapter 7, "Are the Antidepressants Addicting?"). This discontinuation syndrome (should it happen) is not dangerous or life-threatening, but it can make you sick—like a case of the flu. So when you and your doctor agree that it is time to lower the dose or stop the medicine, be sure to discuss the issue of how slow or how fast to taper it down.

Warnings

27

Unilateral Dose Adjustments

MAKING UNILATERAL DOSE ADJUSTMENTS—managing your dose without consulting with your doctor—is one of the two most common reasons why people do not get as much out of their antidepressants as they could. (The other reason is waiting passively for the medication to "do it all"—see Chapter 19, "Aesop's Tortoise," and Chapter 34, "Psychotherapy").

Many, many people do not take their medication exactly as prescribed. There are various reasons for this, not the least of which is that we humans sometimes just forget. True, there may be a subconscious reason, a Freudian slip of the memory, but certainly there are many times when we just plain forget—without any deep, underlying psychological explanation.

Other times, though, patients change their dose intentionally. This is a unilateral dose adjustment. They may take less because they are curious to see if they can do just as well on a lower dose. They may take more because they hope that maybe "more will be better." They don't collaborate with their doctor, perhaps because they are uncomfortable about giving some of their control to somebody else. They change the timing of their doses in order to more conveniently accommodate their personal schedules. They take less because they have side effects when taking the full dose. They take less because they are not 100 percent sure that they want to be on this medicine in the first place, so they "compromise" by not taking a full dose. They take less because of the cost of the medicine.

Such unilateral dose adjustments worsen the odds of improvement. If a patient does not get the right amount of a medicine to the brain for a long enough time period, the medicine is not going to work. Then, when the symptoms do not get better, the patient still does not know if this is the right medicine or not because it was not taken at the target dose long enough to give it a fair chance to work.

Further complicating things, patients are frequently embarrassed about what they did (bypassing their doctor), so they do not volunteer this information to their doctor. Being misled about what really happened, the doctor may then reach the wrong conclusions as he tries to figure out what went wrong and decide what to do next. The following anecdote is an example of what frequently happens.

❧ Case Example

Morry, a retired widower living by himself, came to his family physician with complaints of excessive fatigue, increased sleep, decreased appetite, and weight loss. His doctor's examination and workup revealed no abnormalities except for a textbook description of depression. There was no past psychiatric history or family psychiatric history, and Morry was in excellent health for his age. Morry's physician discussed this diagnosis of depression with him, but Morry did not buy into it. He remained strongly suspicious that his doctor had just missed the true diagnosis. When his doctor recommended an antidepressant, Morry really did not buy into the idea. "That's for psychos and nuts. I'm not a psycho. I'm not imagining this."

Morry reluctantly agreed to try the medicine but returned unimproved several weeks later. At this follow-up appointment, he openly admitted that he had stopped the medication after only one dose, explaining that he had felt more tired after taking it. His doctor voiced his disappointment that Morry had stopped the medicine without calling and discussing it, and reemphasized that Morry could call anytime. The doctor then went through his spiel about everybody being different and needing to find the right dose to match up with each individual's unique body chemistry. "Maybe it's just too much for your body. How about we cut it by one-half?" Morry reluctantly agreed. The doctor called Morry a week later and Morry reassured the doctor that he was taking the medicine as prescribed.

When seen three weeks later, however, Morry showed no improvement. His doctor then recommended that the dose be raised, but Morry resisted. "C'mon, Morry, give it a try. You're not having any side effects on it now, are you? Your body is probably used to it now, and we can get the dose up to where it's likely to work. Right now, the dose you're taking is like taking half an aspirin for a migraine." Still, Morry resisted.

In trying to understand why Morry was so strongly opposed to the increase, Morry's doctor eventually found out that Morry had recently stopped taking it on days when he was particularly tired. Morry stated, "I was afraid it might tire me out even more and, besides, I don't really think it is going to help anyway."

Seven weeks had now gone by, and Morry was still no better. To make matters worse, his doctor had no further idea of whether or not this could be a helpful medicine.

Some reasons for dose adjustments have more merit than others. But however justified the reasons may be, patients should not act unilaterally. See your doctor and discuss the reasons with him or her. Psychopharmacological treatment is a team effort. Do not spoil the team's chemistry by taking matters into your own hands.

28

Alcohol, Caffeine, and
Recreational Drugs, Part II

CHAPTER 17 EMPHASIZES the importance of honestly inform-ing your physician, before you ever start an antidepressant, about how much alcohol, caffeine, or recreational drugs you use. It is just as important to know, after you start an antidepressant, that it's best not to mix these substances with an antidepressant.

Caffeine, even in moderation, can contribute to insomnia, jitteriness, tremors, and agitation. These same symptoms can be caused not only by the "original" depression (or condition for which the antidepressant is being taken) but also by the antidepressant itself (side effects). It is foolish to drink caffeine and thereby increase the difficulty of diagnosing "what is causing what" if you get these symptoms. Caffeine only muddies the water when you and your doctor try to assess whether or not the medicine is working.

Mixing alcohol with an antidepressant can be dangerous. The real problem is *not* that alcohol interferes with the pharmacological activity of the antidepressant, making it less effective.

(Technically, it does not—though it sure doesn't help.) But in combination with an antidepressant, alcohol can have a negative impact on your body that wouldn't happen if you weren't taking the antidepressant: alcohol can hit you harder. This occurs whether or not you already took your antidepressant that day, because the antidepressant has been accumulating in your system. The possible consequence is that one or two drinks could hit you like three or four drinks.

Furthermore, the effects of alcohol can masquerade as, or aggravate, common psychiatric symptoms (see Chapter 17, "Alcohol, Caffeine, and Recreational Drugs, Part I"). So, as with caffeine, why increase your risk of getting these symptoms, or increase the difficulty of diagnosing the cause? If you really wish to get better, is it worth it to drink alcohol and take the chance?

Most doctors advise their patients to avoid caffeine and alcohol when being treated with antidepressants. However, not always. Once a patient is symptom-free and on maintenance medication, some patients are given the green light to imbibe—in *moderation*. Some people can mix caffeine with their antidepressant without any problems, and some people can drink one or two drinks and it will only hit them like one or two drinks. However, if your doctor gives you the green light, you should be aware of the risks before you choose to proceed. And you should be smart enough to stop if you have a flare-up of your symptoms.

No doctor worth his salt will give you the green light to use recreational drugs at any time, much less while you are on an antidepressant. The risk is far too great that the unprescribed drug will either aggravate the psychiatric illness or have a bad interaction with the prescribed drug. Some of these bad interactions can be dangerous and even fatal. Stay away from recreational drugs. They are not an option.

🌿 Case Example

Ben was a gifted guitarist who played in a top-notch rock and roll band. The band had a sizable following locally and had cut two CDs. Local radio stations liked them too, and there were many who believed they had what it takes to break into the big time. But Ben, who was the main songwriter, had slid into a funk, and the band was getting stagnant. At first it was no problem. Everybody (including Ben himself) thought of it as similar to a home-run-hitting baseball slugger going into a slump; sooner or later, he would come out of it. As the weeks dragged by and became months, though, Ben did not come out of it. No new material was forthcoming. Ben's playing was flat, uninspiring, and robotic. He was often late to practice and gigs. Sometimes he didn't even show up.

Ben knew something was wrong. Sure, it had always been hard to get up the next day after staying up until 3:00 or 4:00 A.M., but now he was sleeping his afternoons away too. He had no spark, no motivation. It was like his batteries had run down. Thinking he had mono or something physically wrong, Ben got himself checked out medically. The doctor found nothing but brought up the possibility that Ben may have depression. At first, Ben rejected this possibility, but the doctor's words stuck in the back of his mind. Finally, Ben decided to go to a specialist "to get this depression possibility checked out."

Near the end of the second session, the psychiatrist said he thought Ben's marijuana usage might be contributing to his motivational funk and recommended that Ben abstain from marijuana for a while to see what would happen. Alcohol, which the psychiatrist thought would be a factor, was not, for Ben did not drink alcohol at all. Ben explained, "I don't want to turn out like my father did." Ben's father had been an alcoholic and committed suicide.

By the third session, it became more apparent to both men that Ben was indeed depressed. Ben recognized it in what few melodies emerged into his consciousness—they were gloomy, morbid, and dirgelike. The theme of death continually appeared in his ideas for songs and lyrics. Furthermore, he had come to learn that his inabil-

ity to keep his mind on his work while trying to compose was also a sign of depression. The subject of antidepressant medication came up, and the psychiatrist said he thought it would help. However, he said he would really like for Ben to stop smoking pot before they started any medication (Ben had continued to smoke more days than not in the week before the second and third sessions).

Before the fourth session, the psychiatrist received an emergency phone call from Ben. "I really think I need some medicine, Doc. I'm thinking about suicide." The doctor asked if Ben could see him early the next day, and they met in the hospital lobby at 6:30 the next morning. Fortunately, Ben was not close to acting on his suicidal thoughts and did not need to be admitted to the hospital. But just having the thoughts scared him, and he practically begged the psychiatrist for medication. An antidepressant was prescribed. Ben was informed about the medicine and was again advised not to smoke pot.

Over the next few months, Ben came to most of his appointments on time and proved to be a good psychotherapy patient—when he was there. Once he got going, it was obvious that he was smart, curious, and insightful about what makes people in general the way they are and what had made him the way he was. But Ben had a hard time "getting going" in psychotherapy. He was not a self-starter (at least not at this time of his life). At the start of every appointment, he looked and acted kind of dulled, passive, and flat. The psychiatrist verbalized this observation to Ben, who blamed it on the depression (just as he'd blamed his tardiness and a missed appointment on the depression). "I just can't get goin', Doc. I just can't drag my butt out of bed, even though it's 3:00 P.M. And when I'm here, it's like I don't wake up until you get me going with your questions."

The psychiatrist said he understood, but he still couldn't help wondering if the pot, which Ben was still smoking, was making things worse. Ben got defensive. "I don't smoke it before my appointments. I have never smoked it before I've come here. It's always been at least twelve hours, and sometimes two or three days, since my last toke. Besides, it helps me. It smooths me out. Haven't you ever been mellow, Doc? I've been smoking dope since I was fifteen and it never caused a problem before. I think you need to get me over this depression and get off the pot thing."

The psychiatrist explained (as he had before) why he thought it was important to "take the marijuana out of the equation for now." In the next few sessions, he continued his effort to work with Ben to get Ben over the depression (further adjusting Ben's dose and then changing him to another medicine). The psychiatrist didn't "get off the pot thing" and continued to challenge Ben's usage. "We don't know how the medication, the marijuana, and your brain's chemicals interact with each other. How can we assess your response to the antidepressant when you muddy the waters by refusing to give up your marijuana?"

Ben didn't like this challenge and became quite visibly upset one day when the psychiatrist said he thought Ben was dependent on, and addicted to, marijuana. "No way. I could quit if I want to. I just don't want to. You're barking up the wrong tree, man."

The next day Ben canceled his remaining appointments with the psychiatrist.

29

Interactions with Other Drugs and Food

THE ANTIDEPRESSANTS CAN INFLUENCE other medications you are taking. The reverse is also true: other medicines that you are taking can influence your antidepressant. Such occurrences are called drug-drug interactions and can occur with nonprescribed, over-the-counter medications as well as prescribed drugs. In rare cases, drug-drug interactions can be fatal, but usually they are not a matter of life and death. They can, however, make the difference between whether or not either medicine works and whether or not you will get a major side effect. The following anecdote demonstrates what can happen.

 CASE EXAMPLE

Joan had been shy ever since she was a child. She was probably a genius and regularly received A's on her tests all the way up through graduate school. But as far back as grade school, she'd always been marked down for "classroom participation." No way would Joan voluntarily raise her hand, and she hated to be called on. She didn't

want anyone looking at her and wished she could blend into the woodwork. She was petrified that something might happen and she would end up being "embarrassed to death."

Joan was a loner. She had only a few friends while growing up, and she was not able to get comfortable in a one-to-one situation. She would have liked to have more friends, but that would have entailed being in a group or out in public. More friends weren't worth paying that price.

Joan sat in the back of the room during class, and between classes she slinked through the halls as unnoticeably as she could (still making her A's). She was very comfortable working in the lab amidst beakers and Erlenmeyer flasks and ended up graduating magna cum laude with a Ph.D. in biochemistry.

Her first job out of graduate school was with a prestigious pharmaceutical company, and that is when Joan's anxiety became so bad that she "had to see a shrink" (as she put it). It seems the pharmaceutical company had a "weekly report" meeting every Monday at 8:00 A.M. All research scientists were required to attend and give a brief presentation on what they had learned and accomplished in the week before and what they hoped to learn and accomplish in the coming week. Joan was terrified. "Get up in front of everybody and give a speech? What if I make a fool out of myself? I'd rather die."

Joan had gone to the library and read up on her condition. She correctly diagnosed herself as having social phobia and learned that certain medicines could help her condition; hence her presenting for treatment. Joan had occasionally taken tranquilizers through the years. These helped get her through the situations that she just couldn't avoid (such as defending her doctoral dissertation). They helped calm the anxiety, racing and pounding heart, sweaty palms and armpits, dizziness, and blockage of her thoughts. The only other medication she took was an ulcer medicine, which she'd been taking for several years. Her ulcer was usually under good control, but it would occasionally flare up and cause heartburn, so she took the ulcer medicine regularly for prevention.

The psychiatrist strongly recommended that Joan receive psychotherapy and a behavioral approach to treatment, which Joan politely declined. "No thanks, Doctor. I know about that and I don't want that. All I need is a little medicine to get me through the meetings on Mondays, and I'll be fine." The doctor didn't like this but was willing to compromise for now. Maybe Joan could be talked into nonpharmacological treatment later, especially if medication could help lower her anxiety level.

There were reports in the psychiatric literature about some of the antidepressants being effective at blocking panic and anxiety and in the treatment of social phobia. The doctor recommended that Joan try an antidepressant instead of a tranquilizer, and Joan readily agreed (she, too, had read the reports). She tried one, which didn't work too well and caused her some uncomfortable side effects. She tried another, which worked okay but also caused some side effects.

After eighteen months of trying antidepressants, Joan went back to using tranquilizers on an as-needed basis. She continued to see the psychiatrist occasionally to get her tranquilizer prescription and would smilingly decline every invitation to try a nonpharmacological approach. "I'm getting by," she would reply. On occasion, the psychiatrist would challenge Joan: "Yes, you're getting by, but you're still crippled by your anxiety. Look at what else is out there in life, and you stay in your safe, little cocoon. You're almost a hermit. You're never going to get married or have children" (which the psychiatrist knew Joan wanted someday) "and your clock is ticking." Joan would only smile and say, "No thanks."

Then the new generation antidepressants came out, and in the early 1990s, reports began appearing in the research literature about their effectiveness for social phobia. Joan and her psychiatrist optimistically tried one, and it definitely helped. "I've only taken two tranquilizers in the last six weeks, Doc, and no side effects!" Over the next two years, they tried adjusting the dose of the new antidepressant, and they tried combining it with antianxiety tranquilizers. Eventually, they found the most effective dose and kept it there. Joan wasn't cured by any means, but the antidepressant was working better than the tranquilizers did, and the quality of her life had improved. She remained stable for two years.

One day, she called to report the appearance of daytime drowsiness. She was even having difficulty staying awake at work. "I feel drugged, but I'm on the same dose I've been on for two years. I just got a new prescription filled; could that be it? There's a warning about drowsiness on the prescription bottle."

It turned out that Joan's employer, at the beginning of the year, had offered all employees a "menu" of different health insurance plans to choose from, and Joan had chosen a new plan. She hoped it would save her some out-of-pocket money. This new insurance company had some restrictions on which medications it would pay for, providing better coverage for generic and less expensive medicines. Joan received the same antidepressant when she filled her prescriptions but had switched to a new ulcer medicine. The new ulcer medicine interfered with the breakdown and excretion of her antidepressant, so the antidepressant had begun to accumulate in her system more than usual. After a week, her antidepressant blood levels had become so high that she was having trouble staying awake. Fortunately, nothing bad happened and she returned to her previous ulcer medicine. She had an uneventful recovery and has continued to do well.

It is mandatory that the physician who is prescribing your antidepressant know about: (1) all the drugs you are taking prior to beginning your antidepressant, (2) all the prescription drugs that may be added on later by another physician, and (3) all the nonprescription drugs you may be considering adding on yourself. Furthermore, other physicians and specialists treating you (besides the doctor prescribing your antidepressant) should know about the antidepressant you are taking.

We will not, in this guide, publish a list of potentially significant drug-drug interactions. Given how fast new medicines come on the market, such a list would quickly become out of date, leaving you with a false sense of security that you are safe. It is imperative that you make it your job to keep your doctor fully informed about every medicine you take.

Your doctor will also warn you about possible interactions between your antidepressant and food. The class of antidepressants known as the MAOIs can have dangerous interactions with certain foods. Foods that contain significant levels of the chemical tyramine (like old leftovers and most cheeses), and alcoholic beverages, when mixed with MAOIs, can result in serious consequences. The antidepressants Marplan (generic name isocarboxazid), Nardil (generic name phenelzine), and Parnate (generic name tranylcypromine) are the MAOIs to worry about. Your doctor will give you a list of which foods to avoid if you are taking an MAOI.

The only other antidepressant that has a significant interaction with food is Serzone (generic name nefazodone). Food can delay or interfere with the absorption of Serzone, resulting in somewhat lower levels of Serzone in the blood. This is not dangerous by any means, but if you are on Serzone, it is best not to take it with food.

It does not matter whether any of the other antidepressants are taken with food or not. It is your option whether to take it with food or on an empty stomach.

30

What About Side Effects?

THE NEW GENERATION ANTIDEPRESSANTS are not likely to cause side effects and are certainly less likely to cause side effects than the old faithful antidepressants. This fact is one of the reasons that the antidepressants in general are so much more widely accepted now than in previous years. Nevertheless, side effects can occur with this new generation of medicines. When they do occur, the most common involve the gastrointestinal tract, sexual functioning, or the delicate balance between activation and sedation.

Gastrointestinal side effects include nausea, loose stool, diarrhea, and change in appetite. The effects on sexual functioning could be a lowered sex drive, a problem with arousability or potency, a delayed (or inability to have) orgasm, or any combination of these. Disorders of the activation/sedation balance include restlessness, nervousness, feeling overstimulated, and insomnia, or loss of energy and drowsiness. Light-headedness or dizziness can also occur, as well as shakiness or tremulousness. Dry mouth may also be experienced. This list of possible side effects may seem disappointingly long, but there is no reason to be discouraged: with one exception, the odds of getting any one of these side effects (compared to placebo) are pretty low: less than one out of four.

The one exception is the antidepressant Remeron (generic name mirtazapine), which is the most likely of these drugs to cause drowsiness. Fortunately, this side effect can be reduced by adjusting the dose.

Moreover, there is another statistic that offers the most cause for celebration: the odds of experiencing any one of these side effects so strongly that the drug must be stopped is less than one in eleven. Now compare that one out of eleven with the nine or ten out of eleven who will improve with antidepressants and psychotherapy. This is a fabulous trade-off!

Another point to consider is the fact that what may *seem* like a side effect may not actually *be* a side effect. True, side effects and negative reactions occur with any medicine. But you have to wonder how often a medication gets the automatic blame, when in fact the presence of the medication is just a coincidence. For years, placebo-controlled research studies (see Chapter 4, "Pills, Panaceas, and Placebos") have documented the occurrence of unwanted symptoms when the only "medicine" the patient took was actually a placebo (a sugar pill or an inert substance). So be careful not to jump to the conclusion that you are having a side effect just because you are experiencing a new or unwanted symptom.

Patients with depression or anxiety or panic are especially vulnerable to having physical symptoms, because physical symptoms are a frequent occurrence with these illnesses. So they need to be extra careful not to assume that an antidepressant is causing their physical symptoms.

Also keep in mind that if you develop another illness or medical condition on top of the one for which you are taking the antidepressant, this new illness may cause new or unwanted symptoms. Keep an open mind and consider whatever symptom you are having as just that: a symptom. Then the task becomes figuring out what is causing that symptom.

Even though the odds are against your getting a side effect, anyone can get a side effect at any time, so you need to know about them. Let's say that you and your doctor decide your symptom is a side effect of the antidepressant you are taking. This is no cause for panic. Some patients are so fearful of the antidepressants being potent, mysterious, and powerful that the appearance of a side effect sends them into a panic. They interpret the side effect as a sign of danger and think that the causative agent should be stopped immediately. This fear is unwarranted. Side effects and negative reactions can occur with *any* medication. Even aspirin, one of the most benign and commonly taken medicines in history, can cause side effects (gastric bleeding). The antidepressants are no different from aspirin or any other medication: the appearance of a side effect (once it has been determined that it *is* a side effect, and not something else) needs to be understood and managed. This may or may not mean stopping the medication. Six important points need to be remembered.

1. Most side effects will diminish, if not go away, with time. Side effects will commonly occur when you first take a medicine, or when you increase the dose, and your body is not yet used to it. Give your body a chance to get used to the medicine. Frequently, if the side effect is initially mild and tolerable, in a week or two it will be insignificant (if not gone). If not, then contact your doctor. Of course, if the side effect is major or intolerable, do not wait it out: call your doctor now.

2. The vast majority of side effects are not dangerous. Just how dangerous one may or may not be should be evaluated by you and your doctor. So you need to discuss it with your doctor. Should you contact your doctor every time you get a new or unwanted symptom? How do you know when to contact your physician and when not to? Your doctor and your common sense should guide you. Your doctor should tell you if there are any signs or symptoms that you should call about, no matter what, and that automatically warrant stopping the drug *immediately*. This is rare, but everybody is different, so ask your doctor if there are any such signs or symptoms in your case.

Otherwise, common sense should prevail: if it is minor, not major; if it is tolerable, not intolerable; then (as a rule) do not call. If it is major or intolerable, call your doctor. Minor, tolerable side effects might be slight nausea or upset stomach, loose stool or constipation, slight sedation or stimulation, dry mouth, or bladder discomfort. Major, intolerable side effects might be fainting, vomiting, severe diarrhea or constipation, a prolonged penile erection, excessive drowsiness, or excessive sedation.

It is important to remember that every symptom must be considered in the context of that individual's health and personal situation. A side effect of slight sedation, for example, might be minor and tolerable to an agitated, high-strung, and anxious salesperson, but could be catastrophic for a school bus driver.

3. Most side effects are dose-related and can be relieved by lowering the dose. Everybody is different, and some people are more sensitive to medicines than others. If you get side effects that are major or intolerable, or do not diminish with time, you and your doctor may merely need to lower the dose to get relief. The medicine may still work for you at a lower dose. Do not automatically stop the drug. It is tragic how often a patient will discontinue his medicine and refuse to try it again at a lower dose, thereby depriving himself of the chance to improve on that drug.

4. Some side effects can be put to *good* use. This is commonly done when patients experience some stimulation or drowsiness as a side effect. For example, if the depression is causing daytime fatigue and lethargy, and the medicine causes some stimulation as a side effect, doctors may advise the patient to take the medicine in the morning (see Chapter 22, "Know When to Take It"). Frequently, the daytime fatigue and lethargy improve without even having to wait three or four weeks.

Similarly, if the depression is causing insomnia, and the medicine is causing drowsiness as a side effect, taking the medicine in the evening may help the insomnia.

Some antidepressants are prescribed at night for that very reason: to treat insomnia. This may omit the need for sleeping pills. Side effects do not have to be a bad thing.

5. Some side effects are indeed a sign that the medicine should be discontinued. But this should be a team decision, not yours alone. Remember, one of the two most common causes of treatment failure is the patient's taking matters into his own hands without discussing things with his doctor. Do not make unilateral decisions without consulting your doctor (see Chapter 27, "Unilateral Dose Adjustments").

6. Some side effects are serious, and although you should not be terrified of their happening, you should be respectful of the possibility. However, do not let the possibility of a serious side effect deter you from taking an antidepressant. Serious side effects can occur with *any* medicine. Every year there are case reports of people dying from allergic reactions to penicillin. Yet, penicillin is taken by millions of people every year, and penicillin saves countless numbers of lives every year. Don't throw the baby out with the bathwater. Fortunately, for those who cannot take penicillin, there are many other antibiotics to choose from.

So it goes with the antidepressants (though rarely does anyone die from a reaction to an antidepressant). They, too, save countless numbers of lives every year. And if you experience intolerable side effects from one antidepressant, there are many others from which to choose.

31

What About Surgery
and Dental Procedures?

Due to the possibility of your antidepressant interacting with other medications when surgery or a medical emergency occurs, medical personnel should be aware that you are taking an antidepressant. The vast majority of antidepressants are of minor or no significance at these times, but your doctor, surgeon, or anesthesiologist should know about these to cover all the bases.

The MAOI class of antidepressants (Marplan, Nardil, and Parnate), though, could present a problem. It is preferable to discontinue a MAOI two weeks before surgery to allow it to clear out of your system. Fortunately, in the event of an emergency or a situation in which this two-week "clear-out" is not possible, doctors can quickly counteract any problem that arises. The key is to ensure that the doctor knows you are on an MAOI.

Many patients on MAOIs find it reassuring to always have with them a card that essentially states, "I am on MAOI medication" (and some details about which MAOI). Others prefer to wear a "medical attention" bracelet—the same as some diabetics and epileptics do. In the rare event that they become unconscious or are brought to an emergency room and are unable to tell anyone about their MAOI, such written notification could prove valuable to an emergency room physician or surgeon.

Patients taking MAOIs are the only ones who could have a problem with dental procedures, and the potential problem occurs for the following reason. In order to minimize bleeding, dentists and oral surgeons occasionally inject a second medicine (epinephrine) into the gum along with the local anesthetic (e.g., Novocain or Xylocaine) that numbs the area. The epinephrine causes the blood vessels at the location of the injection to clamp down. A tiny bit of this epinephrine normally gets absorbed into the person's bloodstream, not causing any significant problem because it is such a tiny amount, but the MAOI antidepressants can potentially interact with this tiny bit of epinephrine, resulting in acute blood pressure or heart problems that could be dangerous. Therefore, it is vitally important to inform your dentist or oral surgeon about an MAOI antidepressant if you are taking one.

The solution to this potential problem is simple: once you have informed your dentist about your MAOI, the epinephrine will not be used. Though this may result in a bit more bleeding in the area, it is nowhere near being a significant amount of blood loss. It may be a minor inconvenience for the dentist, but it avoids the possible drug-drug interaction with the MAOI and is worth the trade-off.

All the other antidepressants present no problem, and patients taking them may go to the dentist like anybody else does.

32

What About Pregnancy
and Breast-Feeding?

Do NOT INTENTIONALLY TRY to get pregnant before discussing it with your doctors. Even though there are no significant data proving that the antidepressants *can* cause birth defects, there are also no significant data proving that the antidepressants *can't* cause birth defects. No antidepressant has received FDA approval for use during pregnancy. The fact that there is *possibly* an association with birth defects brings to mind one of the basic rules taught to all medical students regarding medications during pregnancy: play it safe and stop all medicines that are not really necessary. However, you would not be on an antidepressant unless it was really necessary. Therefore, do not intentionally put yourself between a rock and a hard place by getting pregnant without first talking it over with the doctors.

Almost always, you and your doctors can map out a timetable to get you off your medicine (see Chapter 26, "How to Stop an Antidepressant") before you get pregnant. Or it may not be necessary to get off your antidepressant, depending on your individual situation and which medicine you are on.

When medical students ask how to distinguish the medicines that are not really necessary from the medicines that are,
they learn the number one basic guideline to follow—the risk:
benefit ratio. Simply put, do the risks of taking the medicine
outweigh the benefits of taking the medicine, or do the benefits
of taking the medicine outweigh the risks? Applying this guideline to your individual case enables you and your doctors to
make a decision that is best for you and your baby.

Let us consider several scenarios and see how the guideline
of the risk:benefit ratio works. First, let us consider a woman
who has recovered from an episode of depression and is doing
well. She has been stable on the same dose of her antidepressant
for four months. In fact, she is taking the medicine not to treat
any remaining symptoms, but as a precautionary measure to
prevent a relapse (see "Continuation Therapy" in Chapter 25).
She and her therapist have just agreed to decrease the frequency
of their psychotherapy sessions. This was her first episode of
depression. Her husband was extremely supportive of her during the depression and their pulling together not only helped
them defeat the depression but also deepened their intimacy and
strengthened their love for each other. They want to have a
child. The risks to the fetus from staying on the antidepressant,
if she would get pregnant now, would be low. Although there is
not much data on record about the risk of birth defects associated with the particular antidepressant she is taking, the statistics
reveal no significant correlation. The benefit of staying on the
antidepressant is also low. Though she is still in the time period
of high risk for relapse, which the medicine can help prevent,
she has a lot going for her: a history of high functioning before
her depression, no previous depression, very effective use of
psychotherapy, a return to high functioning already, a four-
month period of stability, and a supportive husband. With this
much going for her, she probably would not relapse if her medicine was discontinued. Therefore, let's say the antidepressant is
probably playing only a minor role in preventing a relapse at this
point and the benefit is low. So the risk:benefit ratio is pretty

much a tie, like a teeter-totter with children of equal weight on each end.

What should this couple do? To get pregnant now would either put the fetus at risk (albeit a low risk) if she stayed on the antidepressant or put the wife at risk (albeit a low risk) if she went off the antidepressant. Why take any risk at all? Delaying the pregnancy six to twelve months would be the ideal thing to do. Two more months on the antidepressant would get her through the high-risk period for relapse. After those two months, she could go off the medicine. Then before getting pregnant, she would have another four to ten months to ensure that she is stable while off the medicine.

Next let's consider the scenario if this woman were to get unintentionally pregnant now, with the risk:benefit ratio basically equal at low:low. This would be a tougher call, but the best course of action would probably be to discontinue the antidepressant. It is a toss-up, but the safety of the fetus (especially in the first trimester) would be the tiebreaker; besides, the patient could continue in psychotherapy without any risk to the fetus. And if she were to relapse and need medicine again, the antidepressant could always be restarted.

Now let's consider the scenario of a woman who is going through a third episode of depression. She has attempted suicide before. She has a strong family history of depression. She has improved on her current regimen of weekly psychotherapy and antidepressant medication but is only partially improved. Her appetite has partially improved and she is no longer losing weight (though she is not gaining back any of the twenty-five pounds she lost). What if she asked about getting pregnant now?

Let's look at the risk:benefit ratio. The books list no evidence of risk to the fetus if she remains on her antidepressant (though no evidence of safety either). Therefore, let's say the risk of staying on the antidepressant is low. The benefit of the antidepressant right now, on the other hand, is high. Without it, her depression would likely worsen. She might become suicidal again. Even if she did not worsen, she is not in good enough shape right now to bear or raise a child. She is not eating well, and she is not really able to meet her own needs very well, let alone be responsible for another human being. She obviously should not try to get pregnant now.

But if she was bound and determined to have a baby and did get pregnant, she should stay on her antidepressant, since the benefit far outweighs the risk.

Many factors go into calculating the risk:benefit ratio, and every case is different. Do *not* unilaterally get pregnant or change your medicine without first discussing it with your doctors. Note that "doctors" is plural here. This refers to the probability that more than one doctor will be involved in your care if and when you get pregnant (i.e., two of the following: a psychiatrist, an obstetrician, a family practitioner, or an internist). If one physician is doing it all, discuss it with that physician. Just make sure the risk:benefit ratio gets analyzed by the treatment team and that a good, levelheaded decision gets made.

🌿 Case Example

> *Sherry presented her psychiatrist with the complaint that she was no longer able to get "up," excited about, or even interested in anything. Before this year, she was almost always "up." Others used to refer to her as "the Morning Glory." She had been voted captain of her high school softball team and won a "mental attitude" award in college. She had remained optimistic and cheerful throughout a battle with Hodgkin's disease, during which chemotherapy had rendered her completely bald. After she recovered from Hodgkin's disease and the oncologist gave her the green light, she became pregnant. The birth of her first child was the happiest day of her life. However, nine months later she began getting tired and did not want to do as many of the things that she used to do. It was a chore to cook, do laundry, and take her daughter on walks. Her appetite and weight dropped off, and she began having crying spells. She was jittery and anxious and screamed at her husband over picky little*

things. Family history was positive for depression in both grand-mothers. One aunt attempted suicide, another aunt had received ECT (shock treatments), and excessive drinking pervaded her mother's side of the family.

Sherry's case became more complex as treatment progressed. She did not respond to progressively higher doses of her first antidepressant, and psychotherapy revealed that things at home with her husband were not as happy as they appeared on the surface. For the next two years, her depression vacillated in intensity, at times to the point of suicidality. She and her husband both participated in one-to-one psychotherapy and saw a marital therapist. They addressed such issues as Sherry's new role as a mother and the drastic changes in her life, parenthood, helping each other out, and constructive communication with each other. Furthermore, it came out that Sherry had a long history of self-induced vomiting in order to keep her weight at her usual petite size, and that her husband would periodically drink too much and begin acting like "macho man." These factors were also addressed in psychotherapy. Several other antidepressants were tried along with psychotherapy. Eventually blood level measurements of her antidepressant proved helpful. Finally, her mood stabilized, and Sherry and her husband were functioning well as husband, wife, and parents.

Then Sherry brought up the question of having another baby. She was informed of the degree of risk to the fetus if she were to get pregnant and remain on the antidepressant, and also of her doctor's judgment that the antidepressant was giving her at least a moderate degree of benefit by helping prevent relapse. Sherry agreed with her doctor about the important role that the medication was playing in maintaining her stability. She didn't want to chance going back to the hell she had been through in the past two years. But she disagreed with her psychiatrist's recommendation not to get pregnant now. She and her husband had always wanted two children, she was in her early thirties, her daughter was three years old, and she did not want to wait any longer. The fact that some laboratory animals had some deformed babies after being on doses more than ten times stronger than her dose did not scare her enough to deter her. After all, many other laboratory animals on these doses had normal babies and, more important, her medicine (an old faithful antidepressant) had been in use for twenty-five years and there were no reports in humans of significant risk to the fetus. Her husband weighed the pros and cons in his mind and came out fifty-fifty. Her psychiatrist discussed the dilemma with a few peers, for she—the psychiatrist— was wanting to get pregnant too, and she didn't want her personal situation to unintentionally influence Sherry one way or the other.

After several months of trying, Sherry became pregnant. She had continued to be emotionally stable during the interim, and at that point everybody agreed that the risk to the fetus probably outweighed the benefit of the drug. The antidepressant was weaned downward and she did well until the very end. When she went completely off it, she had difficulty in sleeping. For the next three weeks, she tried to "gut it out," going without any medicine, and her insomnia only worsened. She barely slept at all, and she began losing her appetite and having crying spells. Her husband could not have done a better job of helping out with the household chores and the three-year-old, which she appreciated. In desperation, she took a low dose of her antidepressant one night and finally slept well.

Over the next two months, Sherry and her doctor worked hard trying to get her off the antidepressant. If the crying and sadness were the only price she had to pay to decrease the risk of harm to her baby, Sherry would have discontinued the antidepressant. But she just could not take the insomnia and exhaustion. And furthermore, both her psychiatrist and her obstetrician thought Sherry's insomnia and exhaustion could possibly harm the fetus. Additionally, she was not eating well when she was off the medicine. They finally gave up.

Eventually, Sherry stabilized on a daily dose that was about one-half of what it had been prior to her getting pregnant. She slept well, her mood and energy improved, and she returned to functioning as a mother again. She ate nutritiously, exercised, and did everything she could to provide a healthful environment for the baby developing inside her. She admitted she was scared, and said, "I don't know what I will do if the baby has any birth defects or problems."

Two weeks before her due date, Sherry was gradually weaned down to the lowest possible dose. As anticipated, she slept poorly, but this allowed the blood level of the antidepressant in the baby to also fall downward slowly, which was preferable to the baby's blood level dropping abruptly after delivery. When the big day came, she delivered a six-pound-twelve-ounce boy. He was healthy and spunky, and many sighs of relief were whistled as the news was relayed throughout the circle of family, friends, and medical personnel who knew her. Her son is now eight years old and doing fine.

The gender group and age group that use the antidepressants the most happen to be women during their childbearing years. The dilemma posed by being on an antidepressant and wanting to get pregnant is a serious one, but not an insurmountable one. Women taking an antidepressant should not be deprived of having children, but the timing is vitally important. Careful analysis of the risk:benefit ratio and open, honest communication between the potential mother, father, and physicians are *musts*.

What About Breast-Feeding?

There is not much information on breast-feeding an infant while taking an antidepressant. The available information indicates that, in a lactating woman's bloodstream, some of the antidepressants can be passed into her breast milk, then absorbed into the bloodstream of the infant who drinks this milk. There are reports of possible negative effects on the breast-feeding baby. However, other information indicates that other antidepressants are undetectable in the blood of the breast-feeding baby and that no negative effects were observed in the baby. Taken en masse, what little information is available indicates that breast-feeding safety varies from one antidepressant to another.

Natural breast milk has some advantages over bottle-feeding, and there are occasions when a woman taking an antidepressant will breast-feed her infant. Employing the risk:benefit ratio is a good general guideline to follow. Ask your doctor about both the potential risks and the potential benefits of breast-feeding, which will depend on the particular antidepressant you are taking and the possibility of new information being available by the time you read this book.

33

Cause and Effect

IT IS HUMAN NATURE to ask "Why?"—to try to find a cause for things and to look for an explanation for what is happening when things go wrong. When people get symptoms of depression, OCD, panic disorder, or *any* psychiatric disorder, the same phenomena occur as when they get symptoms such as pain or an upset stomach: they think, "What's causing this?" Patients almost always conjure up at least the beginnings of a theory before they ever set foot in their doctor's office. This is a healthy thing to do.

Unfortunately, it also seems to be human nature to prematurely make up one's mind about what is the cause. People assume that such and such is the reason and are sometimes wrong. This is an unhealthful thing to do and a common cause of partial or total treatment failure. Essentially, they have "blamed" the wrong thing. This chapter describes seven common errors that patients must guard against to protect their recovery.

PARENTS

Patients frequently blame their parents or how they were raised. This undoubtedly stems at least partly from the imprint that psychoanalysis and the various psychotherapies have made in our culture. Yet no parent has ever been perfect. Who couldn't come up with a few examples of how they were "emotionally abused" at times while they were growing up? "Dysfunctional families" are not hard to find. Have you ever met anyone whose family could not be classified as "dysfunctional" in one way or another?

TRAUMATIC EVENTS IN THE PAST

Similarly, events in the past that were psychologically traumatic are frequently assumed to be the culprit. Not many people are lucky enough to go through life without experiencing some emotional trauma at one time or another. Here, too, is "grist for the mill" when people are looking for the cause of symptoms they are having now.

RECENT OR CURRENT STRESS

Recent or current stressful situations are also easy to blame. All people are under at least some stress at any point in time. When symptoms begin, it is only natural to jump to the conclusion that you know exactly what triggered them: this current stress, of course!

AN UNDIAGNOSED PHYSICAL ILLNESS

Physical illnesses are frequently assumed to be the sole source of one's symptoms. This is only natural, too, when you consider how often physical symptoms occur along with the conditions treated by antidepressants: fatigue, weakness, decreased stamina, appetite change, weight change, constipation, diarrhea, upset stomach, headaches, aches and pains, heart palpitations, shortness of breath, numbness, tingling, light-headedness, unsteadiness, shakiness, perspiration, dry mouth, and change in sexual function. No wonder surveys of doctors' offices show such a high percentage of the patient population suffering from depression or anxiety. Not uncommonly, when a physician tells a patient that he has found no physical illness to explain the symptoms and that the diagnosis is depression or anxiety, the patient is skeptical. The patient will fear, or think to himself, that the doctor missed something and that there is indeed a physical illness present that has yet to be discovered.

THE ANTIDEPRESSANTS

Of those patients who do not have an unusually quick and robust response to treatment (which is most people), a few will conclude that the medicine is not only ineffective but is also *causing* some of their symptoms. As listed in the paragraph above, many physical symptoms appear as a result of depression, panic, or anxiety. When these symptoms continue, and especially if they get worse, some patients jump to the conclusion that the medicine is causing them. As was discussed in Chapter 30, consider a symptom just that: a symptom. Do not automatically assume that the medicine is causing this symptom.

CHEMICAL IMBALANCES IN THE BRAIN

Recently, there appears to be a trend to blame one's woes on chemical imbalances in the brain (see Chapter 5, "The Pendulum: Psychological and Chemical Imbalances"). This explanation is flourishing partly because of the astounding discoveries in brain chemistry over the past twenty years. The discoveries have proved that such imbalances can and do exist. However, some of this trend's popularity is because it allows people to avoid taking a critical look at themselves or their situation, which could be painful. It allows people to avoid taking personal responsibility for their problems. Blaming chemical imbalances in the brain is much easier than taking a painful personal inventory.

THE SYMPTOMS THEMSELVES

Sometimes the *symptoms* of a psychiatric disorder are assumed to be the *cause* of the disorder. People suffering from depression, for example, commonly have low self-esteem, feelings of inadequacy and failure, high levels of guilt, and strained interpersonal relationships with their family and friends. One or more of these symptoms may be hypothesized to be the driving force behind the depression. Carol presents a good illustration of this phenomenon.

Case Example

Carol had been a solid B student in high school and had continued to do well in college until this year, when her grades took a nosedive. She had two fresh F's on her report card, dropped out of school, and returned to her parents' home. She'd sleep until noon (or longer) most mornings, then grumble and mope around the house and watch TV in the afternoons. Previously a compulsive exerciser, she completely quit working out. She barely spoke at the dinner table and did more pushing of food from one area of her plate to another than she did eating. Her parents finally persuaded her to see a psychiatrist—the same one, in fact, that her mother had seen some years earlier.

Carol readily admitted to the psychiatrist that she was depressed, and attributed the depression to the fact that she had failed in school and her future looked dim. "You'd be depressed too if you were a failure like me. I blew it and now I'm hosed." Carol also blamed her depression on how she'd been rejected by people who "I thought were my friends. Ha!" She described how they had almost entirely stopped calling her, and she sobbed openly in admitting that she was deeply hurt and lonely. "You'd be depressed too if nobody gave a damn about you."

In her mind, the psychiatrist wondered what had happened be-

tween Carol and her friends. Why did they start ignoring her? Or did they really start it? Maybe Carol did something to turn them off, and she has no idea what she did. The psychiatrist said nothing about this at first and went on to outline a treatment plan for Carol (one that included both a medication and psychotherapy). As treatment progressed, a perfect opportunity presented itself, and the doctor wondered out loud about why the falling-out had occurred between Carol and her friends. Carol was quick to defend herself and was "sure" it had been nothing that she had done; they were just "two-faced bitches."

Carol only needed a few tweaks of her dosage, and she began to improve on the very first antidepressant they tried (the same one her mother had responded to). In psychotherapy, the falling-out Carol had with her friends served as a nice springboard into discussions about how dependent she had been on her friends and others in general. She readily admitted that she'd always been a follower, that she almost always went along with whatever the group wanted, and that her perception of how others viewed her was one of the most important things (if not the most important thing) in her life. She learned about "centering" from within and becoming more "inner-directed." As she improved, her intellectual curiosity began to return. She stopped watching daytime TV and read a few books. Her concentration improved. About that time, her doctor wondered out loud if the onset of the depression had actually preceded Carol's failure in the two college courses, and if her depression had negatively influenced her performance in those courses. "Maybe those courses weren't, in reality, as difficult as they seemed to you, Carol, in your depressed state. Everything looks yellow through jaundiced eyes."

Carol could now see, through eyes that weren't depressed, the possible accuracy of that explanation. At the next session, her psychiatrist again brought up the possibility of Carol unknowingly doing something that had turned off her friends. This time Carol listened. "Maybe I did. I know I wasn't myself there at the end. I just don't know when or how it all really started." They discussed how it would be nice to get some input from one or two of her friends to hear their side of the story.

A few weeks later Carol mustered up enough courage to call Beth (whom Carol had been closest to). Beth said everybody was wondering how Carol was doing and what she was up to, and commented that it would be nice to see her again. Carol jumped at that statement and finagled an invitation to go and visit.

At her next session with the psychiatrist, Carol was grinning from ear to ear. "What a spectacular weekend; and you won't believe this: Beth said, as far as she could tell, I started it. I wasn't as much fun to be around (which I can certainly believe now). Then I started saying that I didn't want to go whenever they wanted to do something. Finally, when I didn't return a couple of phone calls to them, they thought I was mad at them, didn't want to be with them, or was stuck-up or something. So they blew me off. We got it all patched up now, though, and I'm going back next weekend!"

Elizabeth (see Chapter 16, "The Truth, the Whole Truth, and Nothing but the Truth") also went through a form of this phenomenon. Remember how responsible and guilty she felt about the death of the youth who fell off the hay wagon and how it took hours of therapy before she even told her doctor about this. Her "confession" helped her feel a bit better, but she remained profoundly depressed. "Can't you see why I feel so bad, Doctor?" she said. "That young girl died because of me. Wouldn't you feel guilty if you did that to somebody? If only she could be brought back to life, *then* I'd not feel so guilty. I deserve this." Later in therapy, after her medicine was adjusted and she received more psychotherapy, she was able to see how her guilt and the tragic event did not *cause,* by themselves, the depression, but how the depression reactivated and exaggerated these issues from the past.

These cases are tough to treat because cause and effect enter into a vicious circle with each other. The depression causes the symptoms of decreased self-esteem, feelings of inadequacy and failure, guilt, irritability, and strained relationships. These in turn cause the depression to worsen, and the vicious circle just feeds on itself. Like chickens and eggs, one begets another, which begets another, and so on.

• • •

Despite this chapter's warning to guard against making the wrong assumptions about what is causing your symptoms, be reassured that looking for the cause of your symptoms is truly a psychologically healthful thing to do. In actuality, any one or all of the above theories could be the true culprit. Your theory will be a problem only if you are so fixed in your belief that you do not allow for the possibility of other contributing factors. The odds of your recovery will be dramatically higher if you will be flexible and open-minded enough to look at other alternative explanations that could be playing a role.

34

Psychotherapy

O NE OF THE TWO MOST common causes of treatment failure
is the patient passively waiting for the medicine to do it all
(the other one is making unilateral dose adjustments). The vast
majority of patients (if not all) who take antidepressants would
improve their odds of successful treatment if they participated,
at least initially, in some type of psychotherapy or counseling
(also see Chapter 5, "The Pendulum: Psychological and Chemical Imbalances," and Chapter 19, "Aesop's Tortoise"). This
could be done directly with the prescribing physician or with
one of his associates. Psychotherapy can be done in individual
sessions, in a group format, or in marital/family sessions. Regardless of the setup, the patient who plays an active role in his
or her recovery (as opposed to leaning back and expecting the
medicine to do it all) will have a better outcome.

Antidepressant medications are prescribed for several different diagnoses and conditions, as we discussed earlier. Even
when a "chemical imbalance" is the primary culprit causing the

symptom, the doctor or his associate can advise the patient about do's and don'ts while waiting for the medicine to kick in. Gaining mastery over one's symptoms goes much smoother under the guidance of someone who has been trained to deal with these conditions. Furthermore, the doctor or therapist can advise each individual patient about coping with the disorder in his or her unique situation. Everybody is different, and even though many people receive the same diagnosis, the particulars of each individual's case should receive special attention.

Besides, how do you know if a chemical imbalance is the *primary* culprit or not? As was discussed in the preceding chapter, other factors can cause symptoms to appear. In your case, how much stock do you put into the chemical imbalance explanation, and how much stock into the "nonchemical" explanation? Is it 80:20, or 20:80? Everybody has blind spots, so nobody really knows for sure.

Doctors and therapists do not know for sure either, but at least doctors and therapists have been trained in how to help you "take an inventory" and look at the nonchemical factors, and how to do it in a constructive manner. They have been trained to help you tease out what factors may have contributed to the onset of your symptoms in the first place, and what factors may be contributing to the maintenance of your symptoms now. Even then, you still won't know for sure how much stock to put into each explanation, but it won't matter. The doctor and therapist can help you develop the ability to live with the uncertainty of not knowing how much of it is chemical. In therapy, you will address *all* possible contributing factors. Once you have all the bases covered, it doesn't matter how much weight you give to each explanation, chemical or nonchemical.

Certain well-meaning friends or family members will often be there to talk with you, whether you want them to or not. This can be a good thing, for it usually helps to just talk about how things are going in general and to "get it off your chest." This is not a substitute for psychotherapy or counseling, though, for friends and family members have usually not had the training described in the paragraph above. If by chance they have had the training, they should stay in the role of friend or family member and not play "psychotherapist" with you. You need your doctor and therapist to be *objective,* and not be subject to the bias that occurs with a personal relationship.

35

The Significance of Others

FAMILY AND CLOSE FRIENDS should not be left on the sidelines during treatment, as so often happens. Unfortunately, they often remain uninformed, or misinformed, about the patient's condition, the treatment, the medication, and what the medication is being used for. As a result, everybody suffers consequences.

Keeping "significant others" informed about the patient's illness and treatment may seem, at first glance, to be merely a courtesy, a nice thing to do, but not anywhere near as important as the actual treatment of the patient. But it is far more important than that (hence the inclusion of "families" in the title of this book). Let's examine the sequence of events and forces that often happen.

A psychiatric illness always has, of course, negative effects on the patient. These, in turn, have negative effects on the patient's loved ones. Whether it is depression, OCD, panic disorder, generalized anxiety disorder, social phobia, an eating disorder, PTSD, ADHD, or whatever, family and close friends will experience a variety of emotional responses. They get scared. They are afraid of whatever it is that has hit their loved one, of what will happen to their loved one, and of how it might affect their relationship. They get depressed over the situation. And they are angry that it happened.

When loved ones do not understand what is going on, they are not likely to be helpful to the patient. They may think that the afflicted person is to blame for being ill, that it is his own fault. They may believe that the patient could pull himself up by his own bootstraps if he tried harder, but that he is just not trying hard enough to come out of it. They may not even realize that their loved one has an illness. Tragically, about one-third of the U.S. population does not understand that depression (and the other conditions antidepressants treat) is an illness. They think it's a personal weakness and that the person should be able to handle it alone. Such a lack of understanding, of course, has a negative effect on the patient. The patient is bombarded with negative effects from both the illness and his loved ones, who are just adding insult to injury. A vicious circle takes place: without the support of significant others, the patient gets worse, which creates more distress in his significant others, and so on.

Obviously, loved ones should not be left in the dark. Helping significant others to understand the illness, and what to expect in the future, can greatly reduce the negative emotions they are going through. It can't totally eliminate their pain, but it sure can soften the blow.

Once they are informed, loved ones can have a positive effect back on the patient. When they understand what the patient is going through, and how treatment can work, they can truly be helpful to the patient and supportive of treatment. This positive effect will then, in turn, help defeat the illness.

Overcoming the illness is what everybody wants, and bringing family and friends into the battle improves the odds of winning. You, your doctor, and your therapist need your loved ones on your team, part of the therapeutic alliance. The last thing you need is to have them fighting against you.

Unfortunately, we doctors and therapists are not the greatest at bringing family and friends up to speed. Maybe we put loved ones on the back burner because we are so focused on treating the individual patient (talking with just the individual patient, and nobody else, has been the traditional model in psychiatry since the days of Sigmund Freud). Maybe it is because we are so busy treating so many patients. Maybe we intend to, but we procrastinate. Or maybe it is because we have not yet learned the importance of involving them. Whatever the reason, sometimes we need the patient or a family member to remind us to do this. Sometimes we need to be hit in the head with a two-by-four.

Although it is not commonly done, holding a conference "for all pertinent parties" is a treatment option that allows communication to flow, both ways, between the significant others, the doctor, the therapist, and the patient. Of course, who gets invited and who does not get invited should be agreed on by the patient, the doctor, and the therapist before any such conference is scheduled. It is ideal for the patient to be there in order to take an active part in the conversation, as well as to hear what is being said firsthand. Secondhand information, told to the patient after the conference, may lose something in the translation.

Of course, the doctor and the therapist will honor the ethic of confidentiality. Everything the patient has told them in confidence will be kept private. Significant others need to understand and respect this time-honored ethic.

Such conferences are impractical to hold on a regular basis. Designating one spokesperson for the family is a technique that allows updates to and from the doctor, the therapist, and the family. Having a single spokesperson prevents the confusion, omission, or repetition of communications that inevitably occurs when no such system is in place. Communications ideally are done openly and matter-of-factly. Keeping secrets from the patient sabotages the therapeutic alliance, is harmful to the love and trust between patient and family members, and is destructive to the therapeutic process.

36

Relapses and Recurrences

U NFORTUNATELY, SOME PEOPLE who improve or recover, and then discontinue their antidepressant, will have a relapse or recurrence of their symptoms. The statistical odds of getting depressed are greater for someone who has been previously depressed than for someone in the general population who has never been depressed before. Therefore, since the odds of any one person in the general population having an episode of depression at some point in life are one in six, the odds of a relapse or recurrence are greater than one in six. Technically, the term "recurrence" pertains to episodes of depression that return after one year of stability. The term "relapse" is used for a return of symptoms *before* one year of stability has occurred.

If you get depressed again, resume treatment. However, it is important that you distinguish a mild flare-up of symptoms that lasts only a short time from another full-blown episode. A mild flare-up that does not require treatment consists of symptoms that are tolerable and go away after a week or two. A relapse or recurrence that requires treatment consists of symptoms that don't go away after a week or two, or symptoms so severe that you can't wait a week or two to see if they go away.

A true relapse or recurrence should be treated promptly. You do not want your symptoms to get a foothold, which is probably what happened the first time. (As a rule, people do not enter treatment promptly when they develop symptoms the first time. Often this is because nobody realized what was really going on until later.) But now, having gone through this before, you and your loved ones should recognize the signs and symptoms and nip them in the bud.

When a relapse or recurrence happens, the earliest signs and symptoms are often the *same* signs and symptoms that first occurred during a previous episode. Which symptoms these are varies from one person to the next, so you need to look back at your previous episode and identify what your first symptoms were when they first began. Know what your "early warning signs" are, and discuss them with your loved ones and your doctor.

If and when a relapse or recurrence occurs, see your doctor as soon as possible. Unless you are suicidal (in which case you must insist upon seeing the doctor immediately), tell the scheduling secretary that it is fairly urgent that you get in within a week—even if it is just for a quick appointment—and ask the secretary to alert your doctor about your backslide.

If and when a relapse or recurrence happens, do *not* unilaterally make a decision about what to do with medication (see Chapter 27, "Unilateral Dose Adjustments"). It is worth a few days' wait to make the right decision, as a team, as opposed to playing doctor yourself and risk making the wrong decision.

37

Prevention

FORTUNATELY, RELAPSES AND RECURRENCES can be prevented. The most important preventative measures are: (1) Be sure you have, in psychotherapy, addressed all the *nonchemical* factors that could have contributed to your symptoms and that you know and can use *nonpharmacological* ways to cope with your illness and your stressors (see Chapter 34, "Psychotherapy"). (2) Stay on your medication for at least six months of stability (see Chapter 25, "When and If to Stop an Antidepressant"). (3) If you have a disorder that has, on two or more occasions, recurred after your medication was discontinued, stay on your medication long-term (again, see Chapter 25). Similarly, you should talk with your doctor about long-term, maintenance medication if you have a strong family history of depression, if the degree of your depression was quite severe, or if your first episode occurred before the age of twenty or after the age of sixty.

Long-term, maintenance medication for prevention of recurrences is a common practice in all branches of medicine and with all kinds of diseases: heart disease, cancer, high blood pressure, asthma, diabetes, thyroid disease, ulcers, arthritis, chronic headaches, epilepsy, osteoporosis, glaucoma, lupus, AIDS, etc. The list could go on and on. For a variety of reasons, however, people are much more reluctant to take long-term antidepressant medication than they are for any of these other illnesses. Perhaps it is the stigma of having a *mental* illness. Perhaps it is interpreted as a weakness, that you "have to take a medicine" to be okay, otherwise you "can't make it" or you "aren't tough enough." Whatever the underlying cause is, many people are reluctant.

People who are resistant to long-term, maintenance medication are usually uninformed and need to be educated. Long-term antidepressant treatment is no reflection on one's character; it does not mean one is weak or crazy. There is no evidence of health risk associated with long-term use. Maintenance medication is scientifically accepted, effective, and legitimate in psychiatry—just as it is in other branches of medicine. People take long-term medicine for their heart, why not take long-term medicine for their brain?

If certain family members or friends don't understand this, that is unfortunate. They need to be educated. If they still don't understand, do not let their beliefs sway you or deter you from doing what is in your best interest. Maintenance of emotional and mental health is more important than worrying about what others think.

Even with maintenance medication, a recurrence can happen. As is the case when patients take maintenance medications for other illnesses, there is no *guarantee* that you won't get sick again. But, fortunately, such episodes are very treatable. If one happens, you do the same thing you do with other illnesses: go get it treated. Unfortunately, though, due to the nature of the illnesses treated with antidepressants, pessimism, hopelessness, and a defeated attitude are common when these illnesses return. Consequently, many patients feel like giving up. Their depressed view of the world shades their memory of their previous positive response to treatment, and the main thing they see is the fact that their symptoms are back. "Here I am again, so treatment obviously didn't work. Why go back and try it again?"

In actuality, relapses and recurrences may be even *more* treatable than a previous episode. There is now a database of information on what helped before and what didn't. And (we hope) this time the symptoms are being recognized earlier, so quicker treatment can prevent them from getting a foothold. If you do get sick again, do exactly the same thing you would do if you had a relapse of heart disease, cancer, high blood pressure, or asthma: go get it fixed.

38

Giving Up

PEOPLE WITH DEPRESSION are prone to feeling caught in a vicious circle, a whirlpool of negativism that pulls them down deeper and deeper and that seems to gain strength the deeper they go. It can be depressing to have *any* illness, not just depression: to have limitations placed on your life that were not there before, let alone to suffer from the symptoms of the illness itself. So when the illness is depression itself, people get "doubly depressed"—depressed over being depressed.

Fighting depression is hard to do because depression slips into your soul and robs you of your will to fight. Life is not as enjoyable as it was, and you do not care about things as much, so you do not have as much determination to fight. Depression sabotages your fighting spirit and makes it seem like "it doesn't matter" and "it's not worth it." It stacks the deck against you by making you feel too physically and emotionally weak and tired to fight anything. When you fight depression, you have one hand tied behind your back.

Additionally, more salt gets sprinkled in the wound because

of the slow recovery process. Even with up-to-date, effective psychotherapy techniques and more chemically precise medications, the plateaus of no progress and the inevitable dips and valleys along the way make some patients feel as if they will never get over it. Depression seems to exaggerate this by making time drag on, like slow motion. The misery seems to go on forever.

Furthermore, your assessment of whether you can win the fight against depression is colored because your outlook is so negatively biased by the depression. The glass of water looks half-empty, not half-full. It is hard to see any light at the end of the tunnel. The fact that the situation and the future look pretty hopeless makes one even more depressed. The more depressed one is, the more hopeless things look. The vicious circle feeds on itself: depression begets hopelessness, and hopelessness begets depression. Caught in the ever-accelerating current of this vicious circle, coming out of the depression seems like a lost cause.

No wonder it is tempting to give up. No wonder thoughts such as "I'd just as soon be dead" or "They'd be better off without me" creep into one's mind. No wonder that depressed people find themselves wishing they were dead or thinking about ways to make death happen. There is, on the average, one suicide every twenty minutes in the United States. Suicide is heartbreaking for those who love the suicide victim and, of course, a tragic end for the person.

One of the most tragic aspects of suicide is that in most cases there was hope. Rare is the case where there is no hope. Depressed people frequently cannot see it, through their depressed eyes, but it is there. There are more than twenty different antidepressants available in the United States, and over a million doctors, psychiatrists, psychologists, nurses, social workers, and counselors, so do not give up.

Before even contemplating giving up, talk with your doctor about changing your dosage or changing your medication. Perhaps you just have not yet taken the one that is right for you. Perhaps you need a combination of two (or more) medications, a stimulant, or something to augment your antidepressant (sometimes the antidepressant effect of a medicine can be augmented, or "boosted," by the addition of another medicine like lithium or thyroid hormone). Talk with your doctor about such treatments and about ECT. ECT (electroconvulsive therapy, or shock treatments) has a very powerful antidepressant effect. New treatments are being researched while this book is being written and may be available by the time you are reading this sentence. For example, a new technique that holds promise for the future is transcranial magnetic stimulation (TMS): a procedure involving split-second magnetic stimulations of certain brain regions, using a magnet about as strong as the magnet used for MRI scanning. TMS is an outpatient procedure.

Perhaps you are putting too much emphasis on the pharmacological component of treatment and not enough emphasis on the psychotherapy component of treatment, or perhaps vice versa. Before even contemplating giving up, talk with your doctor and/or your therapist about this possibility. True, there is no way of determining exactly how much emphasis you should be putting on each of these respective components of treatment. But progress can get bogged down, or even stopped, if you are consciously or unconsciously expecting too much from one or the other.

Perhaps you are expecting to recover faster than what is realistically reasonable. Remember that starts and stops, peaks and valleys, setbacks and mood vacillations are the norm. Don't give up; remember the tortoise. Though it may seem that your recovery is taking longer than it should, maybe it's coming along on schedule, just like the average patient's recovery.

Furthermore, even if your recovery is taking longer than the average patient's recovery, do not hit the panic button. Almost fifty percent of patients are going to take longer than the average patient, just by mathematical definition. Everybody is different, and some people just take longer than others.

Perhaps it would help to get a second opinion or a consultation from someone else. A good doctor will not be offended or defensive if you bring this up. It sure makes sense to have a new doctor take a fresh look at your situation before you give up all hope. The consultant may see things from a different angle and enable you and your doctor to break up the logjam and get unstuck. Or perhaps you may need to try a new doctor and/or therapist. It would be ridiculous to expect every doctor-patient or therapist-client relationship in the world to be a perfect fit. Certain types of personalities and operating styles just don't match up with each other, and the proper therapeutic alliance does not develop or last. This isn't necessarily anybody's fault— it's just the way the world is—and there doesn't have to be anyone to blame for it. Try to muster up enough courage to address this possibility directly with your doctor or therapist. He or she may well agree with you, and a switch can then be made in a smooth and constructive manner.

If changing doctors or therapists is a consideration, ask different people in our community for names of professionals who are reputable and effective. Try to get details about what makes that doctor or therapist a good choice. Make an appointment and check it out; see how well you match up.

Whatever you do, before you do something desperate, do something different. Get a different doctor. Try a different medicine. Try a different therapist. Try ECT. But don't give up. Suicide is not the answer. Effective treatment is available.

✖ Case Example

The psychiatrist was having a rough night on call. He had already been up all night when he got another page on his beeper around 4:00 A.M. Upon arriving in the emergency room, he was briefed by the intern about the patient behind the curtain. "Someone called the cops and the paramedics after seeing her, covered with blood and staggering toward the river. The ambulance brought her here. She has two deep cuts on each wrist and will not talk to anybody. We pumped her stomach and found some partially digested capsules and pills, which we could not identify. Her wounds are sutured and we are done with her, so she is all yours. She is still not talking, though, so good luck with this one."

She was lying on her side with a sheet pulled up to her chin. At first, all he could see was her stringy and matted red hair. He walked around the cart and noticed her pale face, which still had blood on it. Her expression was blank and she stared off vacantly. Globs of mud had attached themselves to her hair and had dried. He tried every trick he knew to get her to talk, but to no avail.

Eventually, he gave up and told her he was going to admit her to the psychiatric unit under the care of one of his colleagues. Before leaving, he pulled up a chair and sat close to her, reaching under the sheet to hold her hand. He said he did not know anything about her, but he was assuming that she was depressed. He told her that depression was treatable and that she could get better. He said that his colleague would take good care of her and he hoped she would cooperate with treatment. He wished her well.

A couple of months later the office receptionist caught this psychiatrist between patients and told him that someone was there to see him. "She did not say who she is and she does not have an appointment, but she said it would only take about thirty seconds. Will you see her?"

The doctor stuck his head out in the waiting room, and there was an attractively attired young woman with beautiful red hair. She apologized for interrupting his schedule, but said she wanted to see him personally to thank him for giving her hope when it seemed like there wasn't any.

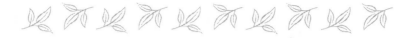

Appendices

The Antidepressants

Anafranil (clomipramine)—One of the old faithful tricyclic antidepressants, Anafranil has been used in Europe for more than twenty years. In 1990 it became the first drug approved by the FDA for the treatment of OCD.

Asendin (amoxapine)—Asendin's unique chemical effects give it a special niche (at least theoretically) for use in treating depression of psychotic proportions (i.e., the patient is not entirely in touch with reality).

Celexa (citalopram)—One of the new generation antidepressants, Celexa has a low probability of causing side effects. Celexa has been the best-selling antidepressant in several European nations, but was not introduced in the United States until 1998.

Desyrel (trazodone)—Available since the 1970s, Desyrel had a chemical structure unlike any other until Serzone came on the scene in 1995. Sedation is not an uncommon effect, and for that reason, it is a favorite of many physicians for use at night to help patients sleep.

Effexor (venlafaxine)—One of the new generation antidepressants, Effexor has a low probability of causing side effects. Effexor enjoys a lower-than-average likelihood of interacting negatively with another drug. It is also FDA-approved for the treatment of generalized anxiety disorder.

Elavil (amitriptyline)—One of the old faithful tricyclic antidepressants, Elavil was the most commonly prescribed antidepressant before the arrival of Prozac. Blood level measurements are a useful laboratory aid when trying to find the effective therapeutic dose of Elavil for a given individual.

Ludiomil (maprotiline)—One of the old faithful antidepressants, Ludiomil is excreted slowly by the body, resulting in sustained blood levels and thereby allowing once-a-day dosing for most patients.

Luvox (fluvoxamine)—The first of the new generation antidepressants to hit the worldwide market (in 1983), Luvox has a low probability of causing side effects. It was the first of the new generation antidepressants to receive FDA approval for treatment of OCD.

Marplan (isocarboxazid)—A monoamine oxidase inhibitor (MAOI), therefore requiring some limitations on diet and extra caution when combined with other drugs. Though not often used as a first-choice medicine for treating depression or panic disorder, it is nice to have Marplan's effectiveness and unique action on brain chemistry in the treatment arsenal.

Nardil (phenelzine)—A monoamine oxidase inhibitor (MAOI), therefore requiring some limitations on diet and extra caution when combined with other drugs. Though not often used as a first-choice medicine for treating depression or panic disorder, it is nice to have Nardil's effectiveness and unique action on brain chemistry in the treatment arsenal.

Norpramin (desipramine)—One of the old faithful tricyclic antidepressants, and one with little likelihood of causing excessive sedation. Blood level measurements are a useful laboratory aid when trying to find the therapeutic dose of Norpramin for a given individual.

Pamelor (nortriptyline)—One of the old faithful antidepressants. Of all the antidepressants, Pamelor was the first antidepressant found to have, and still today shows the most, correlation between blood levels and therapeutic effectiveness.

Parnate (tranylcypromine)—A monoamine oxidase inhibitor (MAOI), therefore requiring some limitations on diet and extra caution when combined with other drugs. Though not often used as a first-choice medicine for treating depression or panic disorder, it is nice to have Parnate's effectiveness and unique action on brain chemistry in the treatment arsenal.

Paxil (paroxetine)—One of the new generation antidepressants, Paxil has a low probability of causing side effects. Paxil was the first of the antidepressants to receive FDA approval for the treatment of panic disorder and social phobia (also called social anxiety disorder) in addition to the treatment of depression.

Prozac (fluoxetine)—The first of the new generation antidepressants to receive FDA approval in the United States (in 1988), Prozac has a low probability of causing side effects. Over 24 million people have been prescribed Prozac, making it the most commonly prescribed antidepressant in the world. Prozac has FDA approval for the treatment of OCD and bulimia nervosa as well as the treatment of depression.

Remeron (mirtazapine)—One of the new generation antidepressants, Remeron has a low probability of causing side effects except for sedation. Sedation is not an uncommon effect, and for that reason, it is a favorite of many physicians for use at night to help patients sleep.

Serzone (nefazodone)—One of the new generation antidepressants, Serzone has a low probability of causing side effects. It also possesses a lower-than-average likelihood of causing side effects of a sexual nature.

Sinequan (doxepin)—One of the old faithful tricyclic antidepressants. Sedation is not an uncommon effect, and for that reason, it is a favorite of many physicians for use at night to help patients sleep.

Surmontil (trimipramine)—One of the old faithful tricyclic antidepressants. Sedation is not an uncommon effect, and for that reason, it is sometimes used by physicians for use at night to help patients sleep.

Tofranil (imipramine)—The original of the old faithful tricyclic antidepressants. Used in the United States for more than thirty years, Tofranil's blood level measurements are a useful laboratory aid when searching for the therapeutic dose for a given individual.

Vivactil (protriptyline)—One of the old faithful tricyclic antidepressants. Vivactil rarely causes sedation as a side effect, and the occasional side effect of stimulation is sometimes used to energize depressed patients during the day.

Wellbutrin (bupropion)—One of the new generation antidepressants, Wellbutrin has a low probability of causing side effects. Additionally, Wellbutrin helps reduce craving for nicotine. The total daily dose of Wellbutrin must be divided up and taken at least six or eight hours apart. It is also marketed under the name of **Zyban.**

Zoloft (sertraline)—One of the new generation antidepressants, Zoloft has a low probability of causing side effects. It has FDA approval for treating OCD and panic disorder as well as depression. It possesses a lower-than-average likelihood of being involved in a negative interaction with another drug.

Organizations You
Should Contact

The more support you have behind you, and the larger your store of knowledge, the better equipped you will be. The following organizations are valuable sources of information and support for people treated with the antidepressants, and for their families. You are strongly encouraged to contact them.

NARSAD
60 Cutter Mill Road
Suite 404
Great Neck, NY 11021
(516) 829–0091
(800) 829–8289 (voice mail)
(516) 487–6930 (fax)
www.mhsource.com

The National Alliance for Research on Schizophrenia and Depression (NARSAD) is a national, not-for-profit organization whose primary objective is to raise funds to find the causes, cures, better treatments, and prevention of the severe mental illnesses. It was founded more than ten years ago by family members and professionals who are convinced that a better future can be found through expanded brain research.

National Depressive and Manic-Depressive Association (DMDA)
730 North Franklin Street
Suite 501
Chicago, IL 60610
(800) 82–NDMDA
(312) 642–7243 (fax)
www.comndmda.org

D/ART Program (Depression/Awareness, Recognition, and Treatment)
National Institute of Mental Health
5600 Fishers Lane
Rockville, MD 20857
(800) 421–4211
www.nimh.nih.gov

National Alliance for the Mentally Ill (NAMI)
200 North Glebe Road
Suite 1015
Arlington, VA 22203–3754
(800) 950–NAMI
www.nami.org

National Mental Health Association
1021 Prince Street
Alexandria, VA 22314–2971
(800) 969–NMHA
www.nmha.org

National Foundation for Depressive Illness
P.O. Box 2257
New York, NY 10116
(212) 268–4260
(212) 268–4434 (fax)
www.ascpp.org

Obsessive-Compulsive Foundation
PO Box 70
Milford, CT 06460
(203) 878–5669
www.ocfoundation.org

Trichotillomania Learning Center (TLC)
1215 Mission Street
Suite 2
Santa Cruz, CA 95060

Anxiety Disorders Association of America
11900 Parklawn Drive
Suite 100
Rockville, MD 20852–2624
(301) 231–9350
(301) 231–7392 (fax)
www.adaa.org

Freedom From Fear
308 Seaview Avenue
Staten Island, NY 10305
(718) 351–1717
(718) 667–8893 (fax)

Recovery
802 North Dearborn Street
Chicago, IL 60610
(312) 337–5661
(312) 337–5756 (fax)
www.recovery-inc.com

Anorexia Nervosa and Related Eating Disorders (ANRED)
PO Box 5102
Eugene, OR 97405
(541) 344–1144
www.anred.com

National Association of Anorexia Nervosa and Associated Disorders
(ANAD)
PO Box 7
Highland Park, IL 60035
(847) 831–3438
members.aol.com/anad20/index.html

National Eating Disorder Association (NEDO)
6655 South Yale Avenue
Tulsa, OK 74136
(918) 481–4044
(918) 481–4076 (fax)
www.laureate.com

Children and Adults with Attention/Deficit Disorder (CHADD)
499 Northwest 70th Avenue
Suite 101
Plantation, FL 33317
(305) 587–3700
(954) 587–4599 (fax)
www.chadd.org/

Twelve-Step Programs

Emotions Anonymous
PO Box 4245
St. Paul, MN 55204

Obsessive-Compulsives Anonymous
PO Box 215
New Hyde Park, NY 11040

Gamblers Anonymous
PO Box 17173
Los Angeles, CA 90017

Sex Addicts Anonymous
PO Box 70949
Houston, TX 77270

Further Reading

This extensive list is offered as a smorgasbord, from which you may choose the references that are most pertinent to you.

General References for Patients and Families

Other Books About the Antidepressants

The Essential Guide to Psychiatric Drugs. Gorman, J. St. Martin's Press, New York, 1990, 1998.

Everything You Need to Know About Prozac. Jonas, J.M., and Schaumberg, R. Bantam Books, New York, 1991.

The Handbook of Psychiatric Drugs. Salzman, B. Henry Holt, New York, 1996.

Making the Prozac Decision: A Guide to Antidepressants. Turkington, C., and Kaplan, E.F. Lowell House, Los Angeles, 1995.

Prozac and Other Psychiatric Drugs. Opler, L.O., and Bialkowski, C. Pocket Books, New York, 1996.

Prozac and the New Antidepressants. Appleton, W.S. Plume, New York, 1997.

Prozac: Questions and Answers for Patients, Family, and Physicians. Fieve, R.R. Avon Books, New York, 1994.
What You Need to Know About Psychiatric Medications. Yudofsky, S., Hales, R.E., and Ferguson, T. Grove Weidenfeld, New York, 1991.

Books About Depression Written by People
Who Have Had Depression

The Beast: A Journey Through Depression. Thompson, T. Plume, New York, 1995.
Darkness Visible: A Memoir of Madness. Styron, W. Random House, New York, 1990.
How You Can Survive When They're Depressed: Living and Coping with Depression Fallout. Sheffield, A. Harmony Books, New York, 1998.
Living with Antidepressants. Elfenbein, D. Harper, San Francisco, 1996.
Living with Prozac and Other Selective Serotonin Reuptake-Inhibitors. Elfenbein, D. Harper, San Francisco, 1995.
Now You Know. Dukakis, K. Simon & Schuster, New York, 1990.
On the Edge of Darkness. Cronkite, K. Dell Publishing, New York, 1994.
Prozac Diary. Slater, L. Random House, New York, 1998.
Prozac Nation, Young and Depressed in America: A Memoir. Wurtzel, E. Houghton Mifflin, New York, 1994.
Undercurrents. Manning, M. Harper, San Francisco, 1994.
You Are Not Alone: Words of Experience and Hope for the Journey Through Depression. Thorne, J., and Rothstein, L. HarperPerennial, New York, 1993.
You Mean I Don't Have to Feel This Way? Dowling, C. Scribner, New York, 1991.

Books About Depression Written by Professionals

The Broken Brain. Andreason, N. Harper & Row, New York, 1984.
Depression and Its Treatment. Greist, J.H., and Jefferson, J.W. Warner Books, New York, 1992.
Depression: The Mood Disease. Mondimore, F.M. Johns Hopkins University Press, Baltimore, 1990.
Depression: What Families Should Know. Shimberg, E. Ballantine, New York, 1991.

The Depression Workbook: A Guide for Living with Depression and Manic Depression. Copeland, M.E. New Harbinger Publications, Oakland, CA, 1992.

Electroconvulsive Therapy: The Myths and the Realities. Endler, N.S., and Persad, E. Hans & Huber Publishers, Toronto, 1988.

Feeling Good: The New Mood Therapy. Burns, D.D. Avon Books, New York, 1980.

The Feeling Good Handbook. Burns, D.D. Plume, New York, 1989.

From Sad to Glad. Kline, N.S. Ballantine, New York, 1987.

The Good News About Depression. Gold, M.S. Bantam Books, New York, 1995.

How to Cope with Depression: A Complete Guide for You and Your Family. Depaulo, J.R., and Ablow, K.R. Fawcett Columbine, New York, 1989.

It's Not All in Your Head. Swedo, S.A., and Leonard, H. HarperCollins, San Francisco, 1996.

Listening to Prozac. Kramer, P.D. Viking Books, New York, 1993.

Living Without Depression and Manic Depression: A Workbook for Maintaining Mood Stability. Copeland, M.E. New Harbinger Publications, Oakland, CA, 1994.

Mastering Depression: A Patient's Guide to Interpersonal Psychotherapy. Weissman, M.M. Graywind Publications, Albany, NY, 1995.

Mending Minds. Heston, L. W. H. Freeman & Company, New York, 1992.

A Mood Apart. Whybrow, P. Basic, New York, 1997.

Overcoming Depression. Papolos, D., and Papolos, J. HarperPerennial, New York, 1997.

Questions and Answers About Depression and Its Treatment. Goldberg, I. Charles Press, Philadelphia, 1993.

Understanding Depression. Klein, D.F., and Wender, P. Oxford University Press, New York, 1993.

What to Do When Someone You Love Is Depressed. Golant, M., and Golant, S.K. Villard, New York, 1996.

When the Blues Won't Go Away. Hirschfeld, R.M.A. Macmillan, New York, 1991.

When Words Are Not Enough. Raskin, V.D. Broadway Books, New York, 1997.

Winter Blues: Seasonal Affective Disorder: What It Is and How to Overcome It. Rosenthal, N. Guilford Publications, New York, 1993.

Your Brother's Keeper. Morrison, J.R. Nelson Hall, Chicago, 1981.

Booklets/Pamphlets About Depression Written by Professionals

Depression and Antidepressants: A Guide. Sen, D., Jefferson, J.W., and
Greist, J.H. 1995. Information Centers, Dean Foundation, 8000
Excelsior Drive, Suite 302, Madison, WI 53717.
Electroconvulsive Therapy: A Guide. Dries, D.C., and Braklage, N.E.
1996. Lithium Information Center, Dean Foundation, 8000 Ex-
celsior Drive, Suite 302, Madison, WI 53717.
Let's Talk Facts About Depression. American Psychiatric Association,
1400 K Street N.W., Washington, DC 20005.

Publications About Obsessive-Compulsive Disorder and OCD–
Related Disorders

Born to Spend: How to Overcome Compulsive Spending. Arenson, G. Tab
Books, Blue Ridge Summit, PA, 1991.
*The Boy Who Couldn't Stop Washing: The Experience and Treatment of
Obsessive-Compulsive Disorder.* Rapoport, J.L. Penguin Books, New
York, 1989.
Brain Lock. Schwartz, J. Regan Books, New York, 1996.
The Broken Mirror: Understanding and Treating Body Dysmorphic Disorder.
Phillips, K. Oxford University Press, New York, 1996.
The Doubting Disease: Help for Scrupulosity and Religious Compulsions.
Ciarrocchi, J. Paulist Press, Mahwah, NJ, 1995.
Funny You Don't Look Crazy: Life with OCD. Foster, C. Dilligaf Pub-
lishing, Ellsworth, ME, 1993.
Getting Control: Overcoming Your Obsessions and Compulsions. Baer, L.
Penguin Books, New York, 1991.
Learning to Live with Body Dysmorphic Disorder. Booklet. Phillips, K.A.,
VanNoppen, B.L., and Shapiro, L. OC Foundation, Milford, CT,
1998.
Learning to Live with Obsessive Compulsive Disorder. Booklet. VanNop-
pen, B., Pato, M., and Rasmussen, S. OC Foundation, Milford,
CT, 1997.
Let's Talk Facts About Obsessive-Compulsive Disorder. Pamphlet. Ameri-
can Psychiatric Association, 1400 K Street N.W., Washington, DC
20005.
Obsessive-Compulsive Disorder: A Guide. Booklet. Greist, J.H. 1995.
Obsessive-Compulsive Information Center, Dean Foundation,
8000 Excelsior Drive, Suite 302, Madison, WI 53717.
Obsessive-Compulsive Disorder: A Survival Guide for Family and Friends.

Roy, C. Obsessive-Compulsives Anonymous, New Hyde Park, NY, 1993.

Obsessive-Compulsive Disorder: New Help for the Family. Gravitz, H. Healing Visions Press, 1998.

Obsessive-Compulsive Disorder: The Facts. DeSilva, P., and Rachman, S. Oxford University Press, New York, 1992.

Obsessive-Compulsive Disorders: Treating and Understanding Crippling Habits. Levenkron, S. Warner Books, New York, 1991.

Over and Over Again: Understanding Obsessive-Compulsive Disorder. Neziroglu, F., and Yaryura-Tobias, J.A. Lexington Books, Lexington, MA, 1991.

Overcoming Overspending. Mellan, O., and Christie, S. Walker & Company, New York, 1995.

Phantom Illness: Shattering the Myth of Hypochondria. Cantor, C., with Fallon, B. Houghton Mifflin, Boston, 1996.

Quit Compulsive Gambling. Moody, G. Thorsons, London, 1990.

Stop Obsessing: How to Overcome Your Obsessions and Compulsions. Foa, E.B., and Wilson R. Bantam Books, New York, 1991.

Trichotillomania: A Guide. Booklet. Anders, J.L., and Jefferson, J.W. 1994. Obsessive-Compulsive Information Center, Dean Foundation, 8000 Excelsior Drive, Suite 302, Madison, WI 53717.

When Once Is Not Enough. Steketee, G., and White, K. New Harbinger Publications, Oakland, CA, 1990.

Women Who Shop Too Much: Overcoming the Urge to Splurge. Wesson, C. St. Martin's Press, New York, 1990.

Publications About Anxiety, Panic Disorder, and Social Phobia

Anxiety. Goodwin, D.W. Oxford University Press, New York, 1986.

Anxiety and Its Treatment: Help Is Available. Greist, J.H., Jefferson, J.W., and Marks, I.M. Warner Books, New York, 1986.

The Anxiety Disease. Sheehan, D.V. Bantam Books, New York, 1990.

Anxiety Disorders and Phobias: A Cognitive Perspective. Beck, A.T. Basic Books, New York, 1985.

Anxiety, Phobias and Panic. Peurifoy, R.Z. Warner Books, New York, 1995.

Dying of Embarrassment: Help for Social Anxiety and Phobia. Markway, B., Carmin, C., Pollard, C.A., and Flynn, T. New Harbinger Publications, Oakland, CA, 1992.

The Good News About Panic, Anxiety, and Phobias. Gold, M.S. Bantam Books, New York, 1990.

Healing the Anxiety Diseases. Leaman, T.L. Plenum Press, New York, 1992.

The Hidden Faces of Shyness: Understanding and Overcoming Social Anxiety. Schneier, F., and Welkowitz, L. Avon Books, New York, 1996.

Let's Talk Facts About Panic Disorder. Pamphlet. American Psychiatric Association, 1400 K Street N.W., Washington, DC 20005.

Living with Fear. Marks, I. McGraw-Hill, New York, 1980.

Master Your Panic and Take Back Your Life. Beckfield, D. Impact, San Luis Obispo, CA, 1994.

Overcoming Shyness and Social Phobia: A Step-by-Step Guide. Rapee, R. Jason Aronson Publishers, Dunmore, PA, 1998.

Panic Disorder and Agoraphobia: A Guide. Booklet. Greist, J.H., and Jefferson, J.W. 1993. Information Center, Dean Foundation, 8000 Excelsior Drive, Suite 302, Madison, WI 53717.

Panic Disorder: The Facts. Rachman, S., and DeSilva, W.P. Oxford University Press, New York, 1996.

Panic Disorder: What You Don't Know May Be Dangerous to Your Health. Kernodle, J. William Byrd Press, Richmond, VA, 1993.

Panic: Facing Fears, Phobias, and Anxiety. Agras, S. W. H. Freeman & Company, New York, 1985.

Social Phobia: From Shyness to Stage Fright. Marshall, J. Basic Books, New York, 1994.

Triumph over Fear. Ross, J. Bantam Books, New York, 1994.

Publications About Eating Disorders

The Best Little Girl in the World. Levenkron, S. Warner Books, New York, 1989.

The Body Betrayed: Women, Eating Disorders, and Treatment. Zerbe, K.J. American Psychiatry Press, Washington, DC, 1993.

Bulimarexia, Second Edition. Boskind-White, M., and White, W.C. W. W. Norton & Company, New York, 1987.

The Eating Disorder Sourcebook. Costin, C. Lowell House, Los Angeles, 1996.

Fasting Girls: The Emergence of Anorexia Nervosa as a Modern Disease. Brumberg, J. Harvard University Press, Boston, 1988.

The Golden Cage: The Enigma of Anorexia Nervosa. Bruch, H. Harvard University Press, Boston, 1979.

New Hope for Binge Eaters: Advances in the Understanding and Treatment of Bulimia. Pope Jr., H.G., and Hudson, J.I. Harper & Row, New York, 1984.

Starving for Attention. O'Neil, C.B. Dell Publishing, New York, 1983.
Surviving an Eating Disorder. Siegel, M., Brisman, J., and Weinshel, M. HarperPerennial, New York, 1988.
Wasted. Hornbacher, M. HarperFlamingo, New York, 1998.

Publications about ADHD in Adults

Adventures in Fast Forward. Nadeau, K.G. Brunner/Mazel, New York, 1996.
Answers to Distraction. Hallowell, E.M., and Ratey, J.J. Bantam Books, New York, 1995.
Attention Deficit Disorder in Adults. Weiss, L. Taylor Publishing Company, Dallas, TX, 1992.
Attention Deficit Disorder: Practical Help for Sufferers and Their Spouses. Weiss, L. Taylor Publishing Company, Dallas, TX, 1994.
Attention-Deficit Hyperactivity Disorder in Adults. Wender, P. Oxford University Press, New York, 1995.
Driven to Distraction. Hallowell, E.M., and Ratey, J.J. Simon & Schuster, New York, 1995.
The Hyperactive Child, Adolescent, and Adult: ADD Through the Life Span. Wender, P. Oxford University Press, New York, 1987.
Hyperactive Children Grown Up. Weiss, G., and Hechtman, L.T. Guilford Publications, New York, 1993.
You Mean I'm Not Lazy, Stupid, or Crazy. Kelly, K., and Ramundo, P. Fireside, New York, 1993.

Scientific References

A medical or psychiatric library is the best place to find these references.

General

Busse, E.W., and Blazer, D.G. *The American Psychiatric Press Textbook of Geriatric Psychiatry, Second Edition.* American Psychiatric Press, Washington, DC, 1996.
Coryell, W., Scheftner, W., Keller, M., et al. The enduring psychosocial consequences of mania and depression. *Arch. Gen. Psychiatry* 1993; 150:720–726.
DeVane, C.L. Differential pharmacology of newer antidepressants. *J. Clin. Psychiatry* 1998; 59(supplement 20):85–93.
Dorgan, C.A. (ed.). *Statistical Record of Health and Medicine.* Gale Research, Detroit, 1995.

Frances, A.J., and Hales, R.E. (eds.). *American Psychiatric Press Review of Psychiatry.* Vol. 7. American Psychiatric Press, Washington, DC, 1988.

Gabbard, G.O. (ed.). *Treatments of Psychiatric Disorders, Second Edition.* American Psychiatric Press, Washington, DC, 1995.

Gilman, A.G. *Goodman and Gilman's The Pharmacological Basis of Therapeutics, Ninth Edition.* McGraw-Hill, New York, 1996.

Goodnick, P.J. *Predictors of Treatment Response in Mood Disorders.* American Psychiatric Press, Washington, DC, 1995.

Gorman, J.M., and Kent, J.M. SSRIs and SNRIs: broad spectrum of efficacy beyond major depression. *J. Clin. Psychiatry* 1999; 60:33–39.

Hales, R.E., Yudofsky, S.C., and Talbott, J.A. (eds.). *The American Psychiatric Press Textbook of Psychiatry, Third Edition.* American Psychiatric Press, Washington, DC, 1998.

Janicak, P.G., Davis, J.M., Preskorn, S.H., and Ayd Jr., F. (eds.). *Principals and Practice of Psychopharmacology.* Williams & Wilkins, Baltimore, 1993.

Kaplan, H.I., and Sadock, B.J. (eds.). *Comprehensive Textbook of Psychiatry, Seventh Edition.* Williams & Wilkins, Baltimore, 1994.

Keller, M.B., Lavori, P.W., Klerman, G.L., et al. Low levels and lack of predictors of somatotherapy and psychiatric treatment received by depressed patients. *Arch. Gen. Psychiatry* 1986; 43:458–466.

Kessler, R.C., McGonagle, K.A., Zhaos, S., et al. Lifetime and 12-month prevalence of DSM-III-R psychiatric disorders in the United States: results from the National Comorbidity Study. *Arch. Gen. Psychiatry* 1994; 51:8–19.

McElroy, S.L. (ed.). *Psychopharmacology Across the Life Cycle: An Update.* American Psychiatric Press, Washington, DC, 1997.

Mendlewicz, J., Brunello, N., and Judd, L.L. (eds.). *New Therapeutic Indications of Antidepressants.* S. Karger, Farmington, CT, 1997.

Myers, J.K., Weissman, M.M., Tischler, G.L., et al. Six-month prevalence of psychiatric disorders in three communities. *Arch. Gen. Psychiatry* 1984; 41:959–967.

Nelson, J.C. (ed.). *Geriatric Psychopharmacology.* Marcel Dekker, New York, 1997.

Perlmutter, R.A. *A Family Approach to Psychiatric Disorders.* American Psychiatric Press, Washington, DC, 1996.

Pies, R. *Handbook of Essential Psychopharmacology.* American Psychiatric Press, Washington, DC, 1998.

Quitkin, F.M. (ed.). *Current Psychotherapeutic Drugs, Second Edition.* American Psychiatric Press, Washington, DC, 1998.

Robins, L.N., Helzer, J.E., Weissman, M.M., et al. Lifetime prevalence of specific psychiatric disorders in three sites. *Arch. Gen. Psychiatry* 1984; 41:949–958.

Rubin, E., Sackeim, H.A., Nobler, M.S., and Moeller, J.R. Brain imaging studies of antidepressant treatments. *Psychiatric Annals* 1994; 24:653–658.

Schatzberg, A.F., Cole, J.O., and DeBattista, C. *Manual of Clinical Psychopharmacology, Second Edition.* American Psychiatric Press, Washington, DC, 1997.

Schatzberg, A.F., and Nemeroff, C.B. *The American Psychiatric Press Textbook of Psychopharmacology, Second Edition.* American Psychiatric Press, Washington, DC, 1998.

Stahl, S.M. *Essential Psychopharmacology: Neuroscientific Basis and Practical Applications.* Cambridge University Press, New York, 1996.

U.S. Department of Commerce. *Statistical Abstract of the United States: The National Data Book.* 1995.

Depression

Agency for Health Care Policy and Research. Clinical Practice Guideline, No. 5: Depression in Primary Care, vol. 2, Treatment of Major Depression. AHCPR Publication No. 93–0551. U.S. Department of Health and Human Services, Rockville, MD, 1993.

American Psychiatric Association. Practice guideline for major depressive disorder in adults. *Am. J. Psychiatry* 1993; 150(4, supplement):1–26.

———. Practice guideline for the treatment of patients with bipolar depression. *Am. J. Psychiatry* 1994; 151(supplement 12):1–36.

Beck, A.J., Rush, B., Shaw, B., and Emery, G. *The Cognitive Therapy of Depression.* Guilford Press, New York, 1979.

Beck, P. Acute therapy of depression. *J. Clin. Psychiatry* 1993; 54(supplement 8):18–25.

Burrows, G.D., Maguire, K.P., and Norman, T.R. Antidepressant efficacy and tolerability of the selective norepinephrine reuptake inhibitor reboxetine: a review. *J. Clin. Psychiatry* 1999; 59(supplement 14):4–7.

Crismon, M.L., Trivedi, M., Pigott, P.A., et al. The Texas Medication Algorithm Project: report of the Texas Consensus Conference Panel on medication treatment of major depressive disorder. *J. Clin. Psychiatry* 1999; 60:142–156.

DeBattista, C., Schatzberg, A.F. An algorithm for the treatment of major depression and its subtypes. *Psychiatric Annals* 1994; 24:341–356.

Eastman, C.I., Young, M.A., Fogg, L.F., et al. Bright light treatment of winter depression: a placebo-controlled trial. *Arch. Gen. Psychiatry* 1998; 55:883–889.

Elkin, I., Shey, T.M., Watkins, J.T., et al. NIMH Treatment of Depression Collaborative Research Program: general effectiveness of treatment. *Arch. Gen. Psychiatry,* 1989; 46:971–982.

Fava, M. Depression with anger attacks. *J. Clin. Psychiatry* 1998; 59(supplement 18):18–22.

Fava, M., Rosenbaum, J., Pava, J., et al. Anger attacks in unipolar depression, part I: clinical correlates and response to fluoxetine treatment. *Am. J. Psychiatry* 1993; 150:1158–1163.

Glick, I. (ed.). *Treating Depression.* Jossey-Bass, New York, 1995.

Grunhaus, L., and Greden, J.F. (eds.). *Severe Depressive Disorders.* American Psychiatric Press, Washington, DC, 1994.

Himmelhock, J.M., Thase, M.E., Mallinger, A.G., and Houck, P. Tranylcypromine versus imipramine in anergic bipolar depression. *Am. J. Psychiatry* 1991; 148:910–916.

Hirschfeld, R.M.A. Guidelines for the long-term treatment of depression. *J. Clin. Psychiatry* 1994; 558:68–69.

Hirschfeld, R.M.A., Keller, M.B., Panico, S., et al. The National Depressive and Manic-Depressive Association consensus statement on the undertreatment of depression. *JAMA* 1997; 277:333–340.

Jacob, M., Frank, E., Kupfer, D.J., et al. Recurrent depression: an assessment of family burden and family attitudes. *J. Clin. Psychiatry* 1987; 48:395–403.

Judd, L.L. The clinical course of unipolar major depressive disorders. *Arch. Gen. Psychiatry* 1997; 54:989–991.

Katon, W., Robinson, P., Von Korff, M., et al. A multifaceted intervention to improve treatment of depression in primary care. *Arch. Gen. Psychiatry* 1996; 53:924–932.

Keitner, G.I., Miller, I.W. Family functioning and major depression: an overview. *Am. J. Psychiatry* 1990; 147:1128–1137.

Keitner, G.I., Miller, I.W., Epstein, N.B., et al. Family functioning and the course of major depression. *Compr. Psychiatry* 1987; 28:54–64.

Keitner, G.I., Miller, I.W., Ryan, C.E. Therapeutic role of the family in major depressive illness. *Psychiatric Annals* 1993; 23:500–507.

Keitner, G.I., Ryan, C.E., Miller, I.W., and Norman, W.H. Recovery and major depression: factors associated with twelve-month outcome. *Am. J. Psychiatry* 1992; 149:93–99.

Keitner, G.I., Ryan, C.E., Miller, I.W., et al. Role of the family in recovery and major depression. *Am. J. Psychiatry* 1995; 152:1002–1008.

Keller, M.B., Gelenberg, A.J., Hirschfeld, R.M.A., et al. The treatment of chronic depression, part 2: a double-blind, randomized trial of sertraline and imipramine. *J. Clin. Psychiatry* 1998; 59:598–607.

Keller, M.B., Harrison, W., and Fawcett, J. Treatment of chronic depression with sertraline or imipramine: preliminary blinded response rates and high rates of under-treatment in the community. *Psychopharmacol. Bull.* 1995; 31:205–212.

Keller, M.B., Lavori, P.W., Mueller, T.I., et al. Time to recovery, chronicity, and levels of psychopathology in major depression: a five year prospective follow-up of 431 subjects. *Arch. Gen. Psychiatry* 1992; 49:809–816.

Klerman, G.L., Weissman, M.M., Rounsaville, B.J., and Chevron, E. *Interpersonal Psychotherapy of Depression.* Basic Books, New York, 1984.

Kocsis, J.H., and Klein, D.N. (eds.). *Diagnosis and Treatment of Chronic Depression.* Guilford Press, New York, 1995.

Kocsis, J.H., Zisook, S., Davidson, J., et al. Double-blind comparison of sertraline, imipramine, and placebo in the treatment of dysthymia: psychosocial outcomes. *Am. J. Psychiatry* 1997; 154:390–396.

Lam, R.W., Gorman, C.P., Michalon, M., et al. Multicenter, placebo-controlled study of fluoxetine in seasonal affective disorder. *Am. J. Psychiatry* 1995; 152:1765–1770.

Lebowitz, B.D., Pearson, J.L., Schneider, L.S., et al. Diagnosis and treatment of depression in late life: Consensus Statement Update. *JAMA* 1997; 278:1186–1190.

Lydiard, R.B., and Brawman-Mintzer, O. Anxious depression. *J. Clin. Psychiatry* 1998; 59(supplement 18):10–17.

The Antidepressant Sourcebook

Mueller, T.I., Keller, M.B., Leon, A.C., et al. Recovery after five years of unremitting major depressive disorder. *Arch. Gen. Psychiatry* 1996; 53:789–799.

Murray, C.J.L., and Lopez, A.D. Global mortality, disability, and the contribution of risk factors: Global Burden of Disease Study. *Lancet* 1997; 349:1436–1442.

Nierenberg, A.A., Alpert, J.E., Pava, J., et al. Course and treatment of atypical depression. *J. Clin. Psychiatry* 1998; 59(supplement 18):5–9.

Paykel, E.S. (ed.). *Handbook of Affective Disorders, Second Edition.* Guilford Press, New York, 1992.

Roose, S.P., and Glassman, A.H. (eds.). *Treatment Strategies for Refractory Depression.* American Psychiatry Press, Washington, DC, 1990.

Roose, S.P., Glassman, A.H., Attia, E., and Woodring, S. Comparative efficacy of selective serotonin reuptake inhibitors and tricyclics in the treatment of melancholia. *Am. J. Psychiatry* 1994; 151:1735–1739.

Roose, S.P., and Suthers, K.M. Antidepressant response in late-life depression. *J. Clin. Psychiatry* 1998; 59(supplement 10):4–8.

Rosenthal, N.E., Sack, D.A., Guillin, J.C., et al. Seasonal affective disorder: a description of the syndrome and preliminary findings with light therapy. *Arch. Gen. Psychiatry* 1984; 41:72–80.

Rosenthal, N.E., and Wehr, T.A. Seasonal affective disorders. *Psychiatric Annals* 1987; 17:670–674.

Rush, A.J., Trivedi, M.H. Treating depression to remission. *Psychiatric Annals* 1995; 25:704–705.

Schneider, L.S., Reynolds, C.F. III, Lebowitz, B.D., and Friedhoff, A.J. *Diagnosis and Treatment of Depression in Late Life.* American Psychiatric Press, Washington, DC, 1994.

Schulberg, H.C., Katon, W., Simon, G.E., and Rush, A.J. Treating major depression in primary care practice: an update of the Agency for Health Care Policy and Research Practice Guidelines. *Arch. Gen. Psychiatry* 1998; 55:1121–1127.

Schwartz, T.J., Brown, C., Wehr, T., and Rosenthal, N.E. Winter seasonal affective disorder: a follow-up study of the first 59 patients of the NIMH Seasonal Studies Program. *Am. J. Psychiatry* 1996; 153:1028–1036.

Shuchter, S.R., Downs, N., and Zisook, S. *Biologically Informed Psychotherapy for Depression.* Guilford Press, New York, 1996.

Shulman, K.I., Tohen, M., and Kutcher, S. *Mood Disorders Across the Life-Span.* John Wiley & Sons, New York, 1996.

Stewart, J.W., McGrath, P.J., Quitkin, F.M., Rabkin, J.G., et al. Chronic depression: response to placebo, imipramine, and phenelzine. *J. Clin. Psychopharmacol.* 1993; 13:391–396.

Thase, M.E., Fava, M., Halbreich, U., et al. A placebo-controlled, randomized clinical trial comparing sertraline and imipramine for the treatment of dysthymia. *Arch. Gen. Psychiatry* 1996; 53:777–784.

Wehr, T.A., Sack, D.A., Rosenthal, N.E. Seasonal affective disorder with summer depression and hypomania. *Am. J. Psychiatry* 1987; 144:1602–1603.

Weissman, M.M., and Klerman, G.L. The chronic depressive in the community: unrecognized and poorly treated. *Compr. Psychiatry* 1977; 18:523–532.

Wells, K.B., Stewart, A., Hayes, R.D., et al. The functioning and well-being of depressed patients: results from the Medical Outcomes Study. *JAMA* 1989; 262:914–919.

Zornberg, G.L., and Pope, H.G. Jr. Treatment of depression in bipolar disorder: new directions for research. *J. Clin. Psychopharmacol.* 1993; 13:397–408.

Obsessive-Compulsive Disorder

Baxter, L.R., Schwartz, J.M., Bergman, K.S., et al. Caudate glucose metabolic rate changes with both drug and behavioral therapies for obsessive-compulsive disorder. *Arch. Gen. Psychiatry* 1992; 49:681–689.

Fallon, B.A., Liebowitz, M.R., Campeas, R., et al. Intravenous clomipramine for obsessive-compulsive disorder refractory to oral clomipramine: a placebo-controlled study. *Arch. Gen. Psychiatry* 1998; 55:918–924.

Flament, M.F., and Bisserbe, J.C. Pharmacologic treatment of obsessive-compulsive disorder: comparative studies. *J. Clin. Psychiatry* 1997; 58:18–22.

Goodman, W.K., McDougle, C.J., Barr, L.C., et al. Biological approaches to treatment-resistant obsessive-compulsive disorder. *J. Clin. Psychiatry* 1995; 64(supplement 6):16–26.

Goodman, W.K., Price, L.H., Delgado, P.L., et al. Specificity of serotonin reuptake inhibitor treatment of obsessive-compulsive disorder: comparison of fluoxetine and desipramine. *Arch. Gen. Psychiatry* 1990; 47:577–585.

Greist, J.H. Treatment of obsessive-compulsive disorder: psychotherapies, drugs, and other somatic treatment. *J. Clin. Psychiatry* 1990; 51(supplement 8):44–50.

Greist, J.H., Chouinard, G., DuBoff, E., et al. Double-blind parallel comparison of three dosages of sertraline and placebo in outpatients with obsessive-compulsive disorder. *Arch. Gen. Psychiatry* 1995; 52:289–295.

Greist, J.H., Jefferson, J.W. *Obsessive-Compulsive Disorder Casebook.* American Psychiatric Press, Washington, DC, 1995.

———. Pharmacotherapy for obsessive-compulsive disorder. *Br. J. Psychiatry* 1998; 173(supplement 35):64–70.

Greist, J.H., Jefferson, J.W., Kobak, K.A., et al. A one-year double-blind, placebo-controlled, fixed dose study of sertraline in treatment of obsessive-compulsive disorder. *Internat. Clin. Psychopharmacol.* 1995; 10(2):57–65.

Greist, J.H., Jefferson, J.W., Kobak, K.A., et al. Efficacy and tolerability of serotonin transport inhibitors in obsessive-compulsive disorder: a meta-analysis. *Arch. Gen. Psychiatry* 1995; 52:53–60.

Hollander, E., and Stein, D.J. *Obsessive-Compulsive Disorders.* Marcel Dekker, New York, 1997.

Hollander, E., Zohar, J., Marazziti, D., and Olivier, B. (eds.). *Current Insights in Obsessive-Compulsive Disorder.* John Wiley & Sons, New York, 1994.

Jefferson, J.W., and Greist, J.H. The pharmacotherapy of obsessive-compulsive disorder. *Psychiatric Annals* 1996; 26:202–209.

Jenike, M.A., and Asberg, M. (eds.). *Understanding Obsessive-Compulsive Disorder.* Hogrefe & Huber, Toronto, 1991.

Jenicke, M.A., Baer, L., Minichiello, W.E., et al. Placebo-controlled trial of fluoxetine and phenelzine for obsessive-compulsive disorder. *Am. J. Psychiatry* 1997; 154:1261–1264.

Jenike, M.A., and Rauch, S.L. Managing the patient with treatment-resistant obsessive-compulsive disorder: current strategies. *J. Clin. Psychiatry* 1994; 55(supplement 3):11–17.

March, J.S., Frances, A., Carpenter, D., et al. Treatment of obsessive-compulsive disorder. The Expert Consensus Guideline Series. *J. Clin. Psychiatry* 1997; 58(supplement 4):1–72.

McDougle, C.J. Update on pharmacologic management of OCD:

agents and augmentation. *J. Clin. Psychiatry* 1997; 58(supplement 12):11–17.

Montgomery, S.A. Psychopharmacology of obsessive-compulsive disorder. *CNS Spectrums* 1998; vol.3,no.5(supplement 1):33–37.

O'Sullivan, G., Noshirvani, H., Marks, J., et al. Six year follow-up after exposure and clomipramine therapy for obsessive compulsive disorder. *J. Clin. Psychiatry* 1991; 52:150–155.

Pato, M., and Zohar, J. (eds.). *Current Treatments of Obsessive-Compulsive Disorder.* American Psychiatric Press, Washington, DC, 1991.

Perse, T.L., Greist, J.H., Jefferson, J.W., et al. Fluvoxamine treatment of obsessive-compulsive disorder. *Am. J. Psychiatry* 1987; 144:1543–1548.

Pigott, T.A., and Seay, S.S. A review of the efficacy of selective serotonin reuptake inhibitors in obsessive-compulsive disorder. *J. Clin. Psychiatry* 1999; 60:101–106.

Rapoport, J.L. The waking nightmare: an overview of obsessive-compulsive disorder. *J. Clin. Psychiatry* 1990; 51:25–28.

Stern, R.S., Marks, I.M., Mawsond, D., et al. Clomipramine and exposure to compulsive rituals: II. Plasma levels, side effects, and outcome. *Br. J. Psychiatry* 1980; 136:161–166.

Thoren, P., Asberg, M., Cronholm, B., et al. Clomipramine treatment of obsessive-compulsive disorder: I. A controlled clinical trial. *Arch. Gen. Psychiatry* 1980; 37:61–63.

Tollefson, G.D., Rampey, A.H., Potvin, J.H., et al. Multicenter investigation of fixed-dose fluoxetine in treatment of obsessive-compulsive disorder. *Arch. Gen. Psychiatry* 1994; 51:559–568.

Turner, S.M., Jacob, R.G., Beidel, D.C., and Himmelhoch, J. Fluoxetine treatment of obsessive-compulsive disorder. *J. Clin. Psychopharmacol.* 1985; 5:207–212.

Panic Disorder

American Psychiatric Association. Practice guideline for the treatment of patients with panic disorder. *Am. J. Psychiatry* 1998; 155(supplement).

Aronson, T.A. A naturalistic study of imipramine in panic disorder and agoraphobia. *Am. J. Psychiatry* 1987; 144:1014–1019.

Asnis, G.M., and VanPraag, H.M. (eds.). *Panic Disorder: Clinical, Biological and Treatment Aspects.* John Wiley & Sons, New York, 1995.

Ballenger, J.C. Pharmacotherapy of the panic disorders. *J. Clin. Psychiatry* 1986; 47(supplement 6):27–32.

Ballenger, J.C., Davidson, J.R.T., Lecrubier, Y., et al. Consensus statement on panic disorder from the International Consensus Group on Depression and Anxiety. *J. Clin. Psychiatry* 1998; 59(supplement 8):47–54.

Ballenger, J.C., Wheadon, D.E., Steiner, M., et al. Double-blind, fixed-dose, placebo-controlled study of paroxetine in the treatment of panic disorder. *Am. J. Psychiatry* 1998; 155:36–42.

Barlow, D.H., and Cerney, J.A. *Psychological Treatment of Panic.* Guilford Publications, New York, 1988.

Black, D.W., Wesner, R., Bowers, W., et al. A comparison of fluvoxamine, cognitive therapy, and placebo in the treatment of panic disorder. *Arch. Gen. Psychiatry* 1993; 50:44–50.

Coplan, J.D., Pine, D.S., Papp, L.A., and Gorman, J.M. An algorithm-oriented treatment approach for panic disorder. *Psychiatric Annals* 1996; 26:192–201.

Davidson, J.R.T. The long-term treatment of panic disorder. *J. Clin. Psychiatry* 1998; 59(supplement 8):17–23.

de Beurs, E., van Balkom, A.J.L.M., Lange, A., et al. Treatment of panic disorder with agoraphobia: comparison of fluvoxamine, placebo, and psychological panic management combined with exposure and of exposure in vivo alone. *Am. J. Psychiatry* 1995; 152:683–691.

den Boer, J.A. Pharmacotherapy of panic disorder: differential efficacy from a clinical viewpoint. *J. Clin. Psychiatry* 1998; 59(supplement 8):30–38.

Gorman, J.M. The use of newer antidepressants for panic disorder. *J. Clin. Psychiatry* 1997; 58(supplement 14):54–59.

Klerman, G.L. Treatments for panic disorder. *J. Clin. Psychiatry* 1992; 53(supplement 3):14–19.

Klerman, G.L., Hirschfeld, R.M.A., Weissman, M.M., et al. *Panic Anxiety and Its Treatments.* American Psychiatric Press, Washington, DC, 1993.

Liebowitz, M.R. Panic disorder as a chronic illness. *J. Clin. Psychiatry* 1997; 58(supplement 13):5–8.

Londborg, P.D., Wolkow, R., Smith, W.T., et al. Sertraline in the treatment of panic disorder: a multi-site, double-blind, placebo-controlled, fixed-dose investigation. *Br. J. Psychiatry* 1998; 173:54–60.

Mavissakalian, M., and Perel, J. Imipramine in the treatment of agoraphobia: dose-response relationships. *Am. J. Psychiatry* 1985; 142:1032–1036.

Mavissakalian, M.R., and Perel, J. Imipramine treatment of panic disorder with agoraphobia: dose ranging and plasma level-response relationships. *Am. J. Psychiatry* 1995; 152:673–682.

Michelson, D., Lydiard, R.B., Pollack, M.H., et al. Outcome assessment and clinical improvement in panic disorder: evidence from a randomized controlled trial of fluoxetine and placebo. *Am. J. Psychiatry* 1998; 155:1570–1577.

Noyes, R. Jr., Garvey, M.J., Cook, B.L., and Samuelson, L. Problems with tricyclic antidepressant use in patients with panic disorder or agoraphobia: results of a naturalistic follow up study. *J. Clin. Psychiatry* 1989; 50:163–169.

Nutt, D.J. Antidepressants in panic disorder: clinical and preclinical mechanisms. *J. Clin. Psychiatry* 1998; 59(supplement 8):24–29.

Nutt, D.J., Ballenger, J.C., and Lepine, J.P. *Panic Disorder: Clinical Diagnosis, Management and Mechanisms.* Martin Dunitz, London, 1998.

Oehrberg, S., Christiansen, P.E., Behnke, K., et al. Paroxetine in the treatment of panic disorder: a randomized, double-blind, placebo-controlled study. *Br. J. Psychiatry* 1995; 167:374–379.

Pohl, R.B., Wolkow, R.M., and Clary, C.M. Sertraline in the treatment of panic disorder: a double-blind multicenter trial. *Am. J. Psychiatry* 1998; 155:1189–1195.

Pollack, M.H., Otto, M.W., Worthington, J.J., et al. Sertraline in the treatment of panic disorder: a flexible-dose multicenter trial. *Arch. Gen. Psychiatry* 1998; 55:1010–1016.

Pollack, M.H., and Smoller, J.W. The longitudinal course and outcome of panic disorder. *Psychiatr. Clin. North Am.* 1995; 18:785–801.

Sweeney, D.R., Gold, M.S., and Pottash, A.L.C. Plasma levels of tricyclic antidepressants in panic disorder. *Int. J. Psychiatry Med.* 1983–1984; 13:93–96.

Anxiety

Charney, D.S., and Heninger, G.R. Noradrenergic function and the mechanism of action of anti-anxiety treatment, II. The effects of long-term imipramine treatment. *Arch. Gen. Psychiatry* 1985; 42:473–481.

230   *The Antidepressant Sourcebook*

Ellison, J.M. (ed.). *Integrative Treatment of Anxiety Disorders*. American Psychiatric Press, Washington, DC, 1995.

Fawcett, J. Targeting treatment in patients with mixed symptoms of anxiety and depression. *J. Clin. Psychiatry* 1990; 51(supplement 11):40–43.

Hoehn-Saric, R., McLeod, D.R., Zimmerli, W.D. Differential effects of alprazolam and imipramine in generalized anxiety disorder: somatic versus psychic symptoms. *J. Clin. Psychiatry* 1988; 49:293–301.

Hollander, E., and Cohen, L.J. The assessment and treatment of refractory anxiety. *J. Clin. Psychiatry* 1994; 55(supplement 2):27–31.

Kahn, R.J., McNair, D.M., and Frankenthaler, L.M. Tricyclic treatment of generalized anxiety disorder. *J. Affect. Disord.* 1987; 13:145–151.

Keller, M.B., and Hanks, D.L. Anxiety symptom relief in depression treatment outcomes. *J. Clin. Psychiatry* 1995; 56(supplement 6):22–29.

Laws, D., Ashford, J.J., and Austee, J.A. A multicenter, double-blind comparison trial of fluvoxamine versus lorazepam in mixed anxiety and depression treated in general practice. *Acta Psychiatr. Scand.* 1990; 81:185–189.

Mavissakalian, M.R., and Prien, R.F. (eds.). *Long Term Treatment of Anxiety Disorders*. American Psychiatric Press, Washington, DC, 1996.

Rapee, R.M., and Barlow, D.H. *Chronic Anxiety, Generalized Anxiety Disorder, and Mixed Anxiety-Depression*. Guilford Publications, New York, 1993.

Rickels, K., Downing, R., Schweizer, E., et al. Antidepressants for treatment of generalized anxiety disorder: a placebo-controlled comparison of imipramine, trazodone, and diazepam. *Arch. Gen. Psychiatry* 1993; 50:884–895.

Schatzberg, A.F. Fluoxetine in the treatment of co-morbid anxiety and depression. *J. Clin. Psychiatry* 1995; 13(supplement 2):2–12.

Thompson, P.M. Generalized anxiety disorder treatment algorithm. *Psychiatric Annals* 1996; 26:227–232.

Tollefson, G.D., Holman, S.L., Sayler, M.E., and Potvin, J.H. Fluoxetine, placebo, and tricyclic antidepressants in major depression with and without anxious features. *J. Clin. Psychiatry* 1995; 13:50–59.

Zajecka, Z.M., and Ross, J.S. Management of comorbid anxiety and depression. *J. Clin. Psychiatry* 1995; 56(supplement 2):10–17.

Social Phobia

Black, B., Uhde, T.W., Tancer, M.E., et al. Fluoxetine for the treatment of social phobia. *J. Clin. Psychopharmacol.* 1992; 12:293–295.

Czepowicz, V.D., Johnson, M.R., Lydiard, R.B., et al. Sertraline in social phobia. *J. Clin. Psychopharmacol.* 1995; 15:372–373.

Davidson, J.R., Hughes, D.C., George, L.K., et al. The boundary of social phobia: exploring the threshold. *Arch. Gen. Psychiatry* 1994; 51:975–983.

Davidson, J.R.T. Pharmacotherapy of social anxiety disorder. *J. Clin. Psychiatry* 1998; 59(supplement 17):47–53.

Gelernter, C.S., Uhde, T.W., Cimbolic, P., et al. Cognitive, behavioral and pharmacological treatments of social phobia: a controlled study. *Arch. Gen. Psychiatry* 1991; 48:938–944.

Greist, J.H. The diagnosis of social phobia. *J. Clin. Psychiatry* 1995; 56(supplement 5):5–12.

Heimberg, R.G., Liebowitz, M.R., Hope, D.A., and Schneier, F.R. (eds.). *Social Phobia: Diagnosis, Assessment, and Treatment.* Guilford Press, New York, 1995.

Jefferson, J.W. Social phobia: a pharmacological overview. *J. Clin. Psychiatry* 1995; 56(supplement 5):18–24.

Katzelnick, D.J., Kobak, K.A., Greist, J.H., et al. Sertraline for social phobia: a double-blind, placebo-controlled, crossover study. *Am. J. Psychiatry* 1995; 152(9):1368–1371.

Keck, P.E., McElroy, S.L. New uses for antidepressants: social phobia. *J. Clin. Psychiatry* 1997; 58(supplement 14):32–38.

Liebowitz, W.R., Schneier, F., Campeas, R., et al. Phenelzine versus atenolol in social phobia. *Arch. Gen. Psychiatry* 1992; 49:290–300.

Lydiard, R.B., and Falsetti, S.A. Treatment options for social phobia. *Psychiatric Annals* 1995; 25:570–576.

Marshall, R.D., and Schneier, F.R. An algorithm for the pharmacotherapy of social phobia. *Psychiatric Annals* 1996; 26:210–216.

Marshall, R.D., Schneier, F.R., Fallon, B.A., et al. Medication therapy for social phobia. *J. Clin. Psychiatry* 1994; 55(supplement 6):33–37.

Rosenbaum, J.F., and Pollack, R.A. The pharmacology of social phobia and comorbid disorders. *Bull. Menninger Clinic* 1994; 58(supplement 2):A62–A83.

Stein, M.B., Liebowitz, M.R., Lydiard, R.B., et al. Paroxetine treatment of generalized social phobia (social anxiety disorder): a randomized controlled trial. *JAMA* 1998; 280:708–713.

Van Ameringen, M., Mancini, C., and Oakman, J.M. Nefazodone in social phobia. *J. Clin. Psychiatry* 1999; 60:96–100.

Van Ameringen, M., Mancini, C., and Streiner, D.L. Fluoxetine efficacy in social phobia. *J. Clin. Psychiatry* 1993; 54:27–32.

Van Vliet, I.M., Denboer, J.A., and Westenberg, H.G.M. Psychopharmacological treatment of social phobia: a double-blind placebo controlled study with fluvoxamine. *Psychopharmacology* 1994; 115:128–134.

Eating Disorders

Agras, W.S., Rossiter, E.M., Arnow, B., et al. 1-year follow-up of psychosocial and pharmacological treatments for bulimia nervosa. *J. Clin. Psychiatry* 1994; 55:179–183.

American Psychiatric Association. Practice guideline for eating disorders. *Am. J. Psychiatry* 1993; 150:212–228.

Biederman, J., Harzog, D.B., Rivinus, T.M., et al. Amitriptyline in the treatment of anorexia nervosa: a double-blind, placebo-controlled study. *J. Psychopharmacol.* 1985; 5:10–16.

Fluoxetine Bulimia Nervosa Collaborative Study Group. Fluoxetine in the treatment of bulimia nervosa: a multicenter, placebo-controlled, double-blind trial. *Arch. Gen. Psychiatry* 1992; 49:139–147.

Grilo, C.M. The assessment and treatment of binge eating disorder. *J. Prac. Psych. and Behav. Health* 1998; 4:191–199.

Gwirtsman, H.E., Guze, B.H., Vager, J., Gainsley, B. Fluoxetine treatment of anorexia nervosa: an open clinical trial. *J. Clin. Psychiatry* 1990; 51:378–382.

Halmi, K.A., Eckert, E., LaDu, T.J., et al. Anorexia nervosa: treatment efficacy of cyproheptadine and amitriptyline. *Arch. Gen. Psychiatry* 1986; 43:177–188.

Hudson, J.I., McElroy, S.L., Raymond, N.C., et al. Fluvoxamine in the treatment of binge-eating disorder: a multicenter placebo-controlled, double-blind trial. *Am. J. Psychiatry* 1998; 155:1756–1762.

Hudson, J.I., Pope, H.G. Jr., Jonas, J.M., et al. Treatment of anorexia nervosa with antidepressants. *J. Clin. Psychopharmacol* 1985; 5:17–23.

Hughes, P.L., Wells, L.A., Cunningham, C.J., and Ilstrup, D.M. Treating bulimia with desipramine: a double-blind placebo-controlled study. *Arch. Gen. Psychiatry* 1986; 43:182–186.

Kaye, W.H., Weltzin, T.E., Hsu, L.K.G., and Bulik, C.M. An open trial of fluoxetine in patients with anorexia nervosa. *J. Clin. Psychiatry* 1991; 52:464–471.

Keel, P.K., Mitchell, J.E. Outcome in bulimia nervosa. *Am. J. Psychiatry* 1997; 154:313–321.

Leach, A.M. The psychopharmacotherapy of eating disorders. *Psychiatric Annals* 1995; 25:628–633.

Mayer, L.E.S., and Walsh, B.T. The use of selective serotonin reuptake inhibitors in eating disorders. *J. Clin. Psychiatry* 1998; 59(supplement 15):28–34.

McCann, V.D., and Agras, W.S. Successful treatment of non-purging bulimia nervosa with desipramine: a double-blind placebo-controlled study. *Am. J. Psychiatry* 1990; 147:1509–1513.

Mills, I.H. Amitriptyline therapy in anorexia nervosa. *Lancet* 1977; 2:687.

Mitchell, J.E., and Groat, R. A placebo-controlled, double-blind trial of amitriptyline in bulimia. *J. Clin. Psychopharmacol.*1984; 4:186–193.

Mitchell, J.E., Pyle, R.L., Eckert, E.D., et al. A comparison study of antidepressants and structured intensive group psychotherapy in the treatment of buli̵ ̵ nervosa. *Arch. Gen. Psychiatry* 1990; 47:149–157.

Needleman, H.L., and Waber, D. Amitriptyline therapy in patients with anorexia nervosa. *Lancet* 1976; 2:580.

Pope, H.G. Jr., and Hudson, J.I. Antidepressant drug therapy for bulimia: current status. *J. Clin. Psychiatry* 1986; 47:339–345.

Pope, H.G. Jr., Hudson, J.I., and Jonas, J.M. Antidepressant treatment of bulimia: a two-year follow-up study. *J. Clin. Psychopharmacol.* 1985; 5:320–327.

Pope, H.G. Jr., Hudson, J.I., Jonas, J.M.. and Yurgelun-Todd, D. Bulimia treated with imipramine: a placebo-controlled double-blind study. *Am. J. Psychiatry* 1983; 140:554–558.

Pope, H.G. Jr., Keck, P.E. Jr., McElroy, S.L., and Hudson, J.I. A placebo-controlled study of trazodone in bulimia nervosa. *J. Clin. Psychopharmacol.* 1989; 9:254–259.

Walsh, B.T. Psychopharmacologic treatment of bulimia nervosa. *J. Clin. Psychiatry* 1991; 52(supplement 10):34–38.

————. Treatment of bulimia nervosa with antidepressant medication. *J. Clin. Psychopharmacol.* 1991; 11:231–232.

Walsh, B.T., Gladis, M., Roose, S.P., et al. Phenelzine versus placebo

234   *The Antidepressant Sourcebook*

in 50 patients with bulimia. *Arch. Gen. Psychiatry* 1988; 45:471–475.

Walsh, B.T., Hadigan, C.N., Devlin, M.J., et al. Long-term outcome of antidepressive treatment for bulimia nervosa. *Am. J. Psychiatry* 1991; 148:1206–1212.

Walsh, B.T., Stewart, J.W., Roose, S.P., et al. Treatment of bulimia with phenelzine: a double-blind, placebo-controlled study. *Arch. Gen. Psychiatry* 1984; 41:1105–1109.

Walsh, B.T., Wilson, G.T., Loeb, K.L., et al. Medication and psychotherapy in the treatment of bulimia nervosa. *Am. J. Psychiatry* 1997; 154:523–531.

Yager, J., Gwirtsman, H.E., Edelstein, C.K. *Special Problems in Managing Eating Disorders*. American Psychiatric Press, Washington, DC, 1992.

Attention-Deficit/Hyperactivity Disorder

Alpert, J.E., Maddocks, A., Nierenberg, A.A., et al. Attention deficit hyperactivity disorder in childhood among adults with major depression. *Psychiatry Res.* 1996; 62:213–219.

Bhandary, A.N., Fernandez, F., Gregory, R.J., et al. Pharmacotherapy in adults with ADHD. *Psychiatric Annals* 1997; 27:545–555.

Cantwell, D.P. ADHD through the life span: the role of buproprion in treatment. *J. Clin. Psychiatry* 1998; 59:92–94.

Findling, R.L., Schwartz, M.A., Flannery, D.J., and Manos, M.J. Venlafaxine in adults with attention-deficit/hyperactivity disorder: an open clinical trial. *J. Clin. Psychiatry* 1996; 57:184–189.

Huessy, H.R. The adult hyperkinetic. *Am. J. Psychiatry* 1974; 131:724–725.

Popper, C.W. Antidepressants in the treatment of attention-deficit/hyperactivity disorder. *J. Clin. Psychiatry* 1997; 58(supplement 14):14–31.

Ratey, J.J., Greenberg, M.S., Benporad, J.R., and Lindem, K.J. Unrecognized attention-deficit hyperactivity disorder in adults presenting for outpatient psychotherapy. *J. Child Adolesc. Psychopharmacol.* 1992; 2:267–275.

Spencer, T., Biederman, J., Wilens, T., et al. Effectiveness and tolerability of tomoxetine in adults with attention deficit hyperactivity disorder. *Am. J. Psychiatry* 1998; 155:693–695.

Wender, P.H., and Reimherr, F.W. Bupropion treatment of attention deficit hyperactivity disorder in adults. *Am. J. Psychiatry* 1990; 147:1018–1020.

Wender, P.H., Wood, D.R., and Reimherr, F.W. Pharmacological treatment of attention deficit disorder residual type (ADD, RT, "minimal brain dysfunction," "hyperactivity") in adults. *Psychopharmacol. Bull.* 1985; 21:222–230.

Wender, P.H., Wood, D.R., Reimherr, F.W., Ward, M. An open trial of pargyline in the treatment of attention deficit disorder, residual type. *Psychiatry Res.* 1983; 9:329–336.

Wilens, T.E., Biederman, J., Mick, E., and Spencer, T. A systematic assessment of tricyclic antidepressants in the treatment of adult attention-deficit hyperactivity disorder. *J. Nerv. Ment. Dis.* 1995; 183:48–50.

Wilens, T.E., Biederman, J., Prince, J., et al. Six week, double-blind, placebo-controlled study of desipramine for adult attention deficit hyperactivity disorder. *Am. J. Psychiatry* 1996; 153:1147–1153.

Wilens, T.E., Biederman, J., Spencer, T.J., and Prince, J. Pharmacotherapy of adult attention deficit/hyperactivity disorder: a review. *J. Clin. Psychopharmacol.* 1995; 15:270–279.

Post-Traumatic Stress Disorder

Burstein, A. Treatment of post-traumatic stress disorder with imipramine. *Psychosomatics* 1984; 25:681–687.

Davidson, J.R.T. Drug therapy of post-traumatic stress disorder. *Br. J. Psychiatry* 1992; 160:309–314.

Davidson, J.R.T., Kudler, H., Smith, R., et al. Treatment of posttraumatic stress disorder with amitriptyline and placebo. *Arch. Gen. Psychiatry* 1990; 47:259–266.

Davidson, J.R.T., Roth, S., and Newan, E. Treatment of post traumatic stress disorder with fluoxetine. *J. Traumatic Stress* 1991; 4:419–423.

Frank, J.B., Kosten, T.R., Gilles, E.L., et al. A randomized clinical trial of phenelzine and imipramine for posttraumatic stress disorder. *Am. J. Psychiatry* 1988; 145:1289–1291.

Freidy, J.R., and Hobfoll, S.E. (eds.). *Traumatic Stress*. Plenum Press, New York, 1996.

Friedman, M.J. Toward rational pharmacotherapy for posttraumatic stress disorder: an interim report. *Am. J. Psychiatry* 1988; 145:281–285.

————. Biological approaches to the diagnosis and treatment of post traumatic stress disorder. *J. Traumatic Stress* 1991; 4:67–91.

Hertzberg, M.A., Feldman, M.E., Beckham, J.C., and Davidson, J.R.T. Trial of trazodone for posttraumatic stress disorder using a multiple baseline group design. *J. Clin. Psychopharmacol.* 1996; 16:294–298.

Kline, N.A., Dow, B.M., Brown, S.A., and Matloff, J.L. Sertraline efficacy in depressed combat veterans with posttraumatic stress disorder. *Am. J. Psychiatry* 1994; 151:621.

Kosten, T.R., Frank, J.B., Dan, E., et al. Pharmacotherapy for post traumatic stress disorder using phenelzine and imipramine. *J. Nerv. Ment. Dis.* 1991; 179:366–370.

Marmar, C.R., Schoenfeld, F., Weiss, D.S., et al. Open trial of fluoxetine treatment for combat-related posttraumatic stress disorder. *J. Clin. Psychiatry* 1996; 57(supplement 8):66–72.

Marshall, R.D., Klein, D.F. Pharmacotherapy in the treatment of posttraumatic stress disorder. *Psychiatric Annals* 1995; 25:588–597.

Marshall, R.D., Stein, D.J., Liebowitz, M.R., and Yehuda, R. A pharmacotherapy algorithm in the treatment of posttraumatic stress disorder. *Psychiatric Annals* 1996; 26:217–226.

Mirabella, R.F., Frueh, B.C., and Fossey, M.D. Exposure therapy and antidepressant medication for treatment of chronic PTSD. *Am. J. Psychiatry* 1995; 152:955–956.

Nagy, L.M., Morgan, C.A., Southwick, S.M., et al. Open prospective trial of fluoxetine for posttraumatic stress disorder. *J. Clin. Psychopharmacol.* 1991; 13:107–113.

Solomon, S.D., Gerrity, E.T., and Muff, A.M. Efficacy of treatments for posttraumatic stress disorder: an empirical review. *JAMA* 1992; 268:633–638.

VanderKolk, B.A., Dreyfuss, D., Michaels, M., et al. Fluoxetine in posttraumatic stress disorder. *J. Clin. Psychiatry* 1994; 55:517–522.

Obsessive-Compulsive Related Disorders

Hollander, E. *Obsessive-Compulsive Related Disorders*. American Psychiatric Press, Washington, DC, 1993.

————. Obsessive-Compulsive spectrum disorders: an overview. *Psychiatric Annals* 1993; 23:355–358.

Hollander, E., Kuvon, J.H., Stein, D.J., et al. Obsessive-compulsive and spectrum disorders: overview and quality of life issues. *J. Clin. Psychiatry* 1996; 57(supplement 8):3–6.

Hollander, E., and Long, C.M. Obsessive-compulsive spectrum disorders. *J. Clin. Psychiatry* 1995; 56(supplement 4):3–6.

McElroy, S.L., Hudson, J.I., Pope, H.E. Jr., et al. The DSM III-R impulse control disorders not elsewhere classified: clinical characteristics and relationship to other psychiatric disorders. *Am. J. Psychiatry* 1992; 149:318–327.

Oldham, J.M., Hollander, E., and Skodol, A.E. (eds.). *Impulsivity and Compulsivity*. American Psychiatric Press, Washington, DC, 1996.

Simeon, D., Stein, D.J., Gross, S., et al. A double-blind trial of fluoxetine in pathologic skin picking. *J. Clin. Psychiatry* 1997; 58:341–347.

Yaryura-Tobias, J.A., Neziroglu, F.A. *Obsessive-Compulsive Disorder Spectrum: Pathogenesis, Diagnosis, and Treatment*. American Psychiatric Press, Washington, DC, 1996.

Trichotillomania

Christenson, G.A., and Crow, S.J. The characterization and treatment of trichotillomania. *J. Clin. Psychiatry* 1996; 57(supplement 8):42–44.

Christenson, G.A., MacKenzie, T.B., and Mitchell, J.E. Characteristics of 60 adult chronic hair pullers. *Am. J. Psychiatry* 1991; 148:365–370.

Cohen, L.J., Stein, D.J., Simeon, D., et al. Clinical profile, comorbidity, and treatment history in 123 hair pullers: a survey study. *J. Clin. Psychiatry* 1995; 56:319–326.

Jaspers, J.P.C. The diagnosis and psychopharmacological treatment of trichotillomania: a review. *Pharmacopsychiatry* 1996; 29:115–120.

Keuthen, N.J., O'Sullivan, R.L., Goodchild, P., et al. Retrospective review of treatment outcome for 63 patients with trichotillomania. *Am. J. Psychiatry* 1998; 155:560–561.

O'Sullivan, R.L., Keuthen, N.J., Christenson, G.A., et al. Trichotillomania: behavioral symptom or clinical syndrome? *Am. J. Psychiatry* 1997; 154:1442–1449.

Steichenwein, S.M., and Thornby, J.I. A long-term placebo-controlled crossover trial of the efficacy of fluoxetine for trichotillomania. *Am. J. Psychiatry* 1995; 152:1192–1196.

Swedo, S. Trichotillomania. *Psychiatric Annals* 1993; 23:402–407.

Swedo, S.E., Lenane, M.C., and Leonard, H.L. Long-term treatment of trichotillomania. *N. Engl. J. Med.* 1993; 329:141–142.

Swedo, S.E., and Leonard, L.L. Trichotillomania: an obsessive-compulsive spectrum disorder? *Psychiatric Clin. North Am.* 1992; 15:777–790.

Swedo, S.E., Leonard, H.L., Rapoport, J.L., et al. A double-blind comparison of clomipramine and desipramine in treatment of trichotillomania (hair pulling). *N. Engl. J. Med.* 1989; 321:497–501.

Winchel, R.M. Trichotillomania: presentation and treatment. *Psychiatric Annals* 1992; 22:84–89.

Body Dysmorphic Disorder

Hollander, E., Cohen, L.J., and Simeon, D. Body dysmorphic disorder. *Psychiatric Annals* 1993; 23:359–364.

Hollander, E., Cohen, L.J., Simeon, D., et al. Fluvoxamine treatment of body dysmorphic disorder. *J. Clin. Psychopharmacol.* 1994; 14:75–77.

Hollander, E., Liebowitz, M.R., Winchel, R., et al. Treatment of body dysmorphic disorder with serotonin reuptake blockers. *Am. J. Psychiatry* 1989; 146:768–770.

Phillips, K.A. Body dysmorphic disorder: clinical features and drug treatment. *CNS Drugs* 1995; 3:30–40.

———. Body dysmorphic disorder: diagnosis and treatment of imagined ugliness. *J. Clin. Psychiatry* 1996; 57(supplement 8):61–65.

Phillips, K.A., McElroy, S.L., Keck, P.E. Jr., et al. Body dysmorphic disorder: thirty cases of imagined ugliness. *Am. J. Psychiatry* 1993; 150:302–308.

Phillips, K.A., McElroy, S.L., Keck, P.E. Jr., et al. A comparison of delusional and non-delusional body dysmorphic disorder in 100 cases. *Psychopharmacol. Bull.* 1994; 30:179–186.

Hypochondriasis

Fallon, B.A., Javitch, J.A., Hollander, E., and Liebowitz, M.R. Hypochondriasis and obsessive-compulsive disorder: overlaps in diagnosis and treatment. *J. Clin. Psychiatry* 1991; 52:457–460.

Fallon, B.A., Klein, B.W., and Liebowitz, M.R. Hypochondriasis: treatment strategies. *Psychiatric Annals* 1993; 23:374–381.

Fallon, B.A., Leibowitz, M.R., Salman, E., et al. Fluoxetine for hypochondriacal patients without major depression. *J. Clin. Psychopharmacol.* 1993; 13:438–441.

Viswanathan, R., and Paradis, C. Treatment of cancer phobia with fluoxetine. *Am. J. Psychiatry* 1991; 148:4090.

Wenner, R.B., Noyes, R. Imipramine: an effective treatment for illness phobia. *J. Affect. Disord.* 1991; 22:43–48.

Depersonalization Disorder

Abbas, S., Chandra, P., and Srivastava, M. The use of fluoxetine and buspirone for treatment-refractory depersonalization disorder. *J. Clin. Psychiatry* 1995; 56:484–493.

Fichtner, C.G., Horevitz, R.P., and Braun, B.G. Fluoxetine in depersonalization disorder. *Am. J. Psychiatry* 1992; 149:1750–1751.

Hollander, E., Liebowitz, M.R., DeCaria, C., et al. Treatment of depersonalization with serotonin reuptake blockers. *J. Clin. Psychiatry* 1990; 10:200–203.

Ratliff, N.B., and Kerski, D. Depersonalization treated with fluoxetine. *Am. J. Psychiatry* 1995; 152:1689–1690.

Simeon, D., Gross, S., Guralnik, C.D., et al. Feeling unreal: 30 cases of DSM-III-R depersonalization disorder. *Am. J. Psychiatry* 1997; 154:1107–1113.

Simeon, D., Hollander, E. Depersonalization disorder. *Psychiatric Annals* 1993; 23:382–388.

Kleptomania

Fishbain, D.A. Kleptomania as a risk-taking behavior in response to depression. *Am. J. Psychother.* 1987; 41:598–603.

Goldman, M.J. Kleptomania: making sense of the nonsensical. *Am. J. Psychiatry* 1991; 148:986–996.

McElroy, S.L., Keck, P.E., Phillips, K.A. Kleptomania, compulsive buying, and binge eating disorder. *J. Clin. Psychiatry* 1995; 56(supplement 4):14–26.

McElroy, S.L., Keck, P.E. Jr., Pulp, H.G. Jr., et al. Pharmacological treatment of kleptomania and bulimia nervosa. *J. Clin. Psychopharmacol.* 1989; 9:358–360.

McElroy, S.L., Pope, H.G. Jr., Hudson, J.I., et al. Kleptomania: a report of 20 cases. *Am. J. Psychiatry* 1991; 148:652–657.

Pathological Gambling

Blanco, C., Orensanz-Munoz, L., Blanco-Jerez, C., et al. Pathological gambling and platelet MAO activity: a psychobiological study. *Am. J. Psychiatry* 1996; 153:119–121.

Cartwright, C., DeCaria, C.M., and Hollander, E. Pathological gambling: a clinical review. *J. Prac. Psych. and Behav. Health* 1998; 4:277–286.

DeCaria, C.M., Hollander, E., Grossman, R., et al. Diagnosis, neurobiology and treatment of pathological gambling. *J. Clin. Psychiatry* 1996; 57:80–84.

Hollander, E., Begaz, T., and DeCaria, C.M. Pharmacologic approaches in the treatment of pathologic gambling. *CNS Spectrums* 1998; 6:72–80.

Hollander, E., DeCaria, C., Mari, E.M., et al. Short-term single-blind fluvoxamine treatment of pathologic gambling. *Am. J. Psychiatry* 1998; 155:1781–1783.

Hollander, E., Frenkel, M., DeCaria, C., et al. Treatment of pathological gambling with clomipramine. *Am. J. Psychiatry* 1992; 149:710–711.

Roy, A., Adinoff, B., Roehrich, L., et al. Pathological gambling: a psychobiological study. *Arch. Gen. Psychiatry* 1988; 45:369–373.

Sexual Addictions

Bianci, M.D. Fluoxetine treatment of exhibitionism. *Am. J. Psychiatry* 1990; 147:1089–1090.

Black, D.W. Compulsive sexual behavior: a review. *J. Prac. Psych. and Behav. Health* 1998; 4:219–229.

Emmanuel, N.P., Lydiard, R.B., and Ballenger, J.C. Fluoxetine treatment of voyeurism. *Am. J. Psychiatry* 1991; 148:950.

Stein, D.J., Hollander, E., Anthony, D.T., et al. Serotonergic medications for sexual obsessions, sexual addictions, and paraphilias. *J. Clin. Psychiatry* 1992; 53:267–271.

Compulsive Buying

Black, D.W. Compulsive buying: a review. *J. Clin. Psychiatry* 1996; 57(supplement 8):50–55.

Christenson, G.A., Faber, R.J., deZwaan, M., et al. Compulsive buying: descriptive characteristics and psychiatric comorbidity. *J. Clin. Psychiatry* 1994; 55:5–11.

Lejoyeux, M., Ades, J., Tassain, V., and Solomon, J. Phenomenology and psychopathology of uncontrolled buying. *Am. J. Psychiatry* 1996; 153:1524–1529.

Lejoyeux, M., Hortane, M., and Ades, J. Compulsive buying and depression. *J. Clin. Psychiatry* 1995; 56:38.

McElroy, S.L., Keck, P.E. Jr., Pope, H.G. Jr., et al. Compulsive buying: a report of 20 cases. *J. Clin. Psychiatry* 1994; 55:242–248.

McElroy, S.L., Satlin, A., Pope, H.G. Jr., et al. Treatment of compulsive shopping with antidepressants: a report of 3 cases. *Ann. Clin. Psychiatry* 1991; 3:199–204.

Premenstrual Dysphoric Disorder

Freeman, E.W., Rickels, K., and Sondheimer, S.J. Fluvoxamine for premenstrual dysphoria: a pilot study. *J. Clin. Psychiatry* 1996; 57(supplement 8):56–60.

Freeman, E.W., Rickels, K., Sondheimer, S.J., et al. Nefazodone in the treatment of premenstrual syndrome: a preliminary study. *J. Clin. Psychopharmacol.* 1994; 16:180–186.

Pearlstone, T.B., and Stone, A.B. Long-term fluoxetine treatment of late luteal phase dysphoric disorder. *J. Clin. Psychiatry* 1994; 55:332–335.

Pearlstein, T.B., Stone, A.B., Lund, S.A., et al. Comparison of fluoxetine, buproprion, and placebo in the treatment of premenstrual dysphoric disorder. *J. Clin. Psychopharmacol.* 1998; 17:261–266.

Steiner, M., Steinberg, S., Stewart, D., et al. Fluoxetine in the treatment of premenstrual dysphoria. *N. Engl. J. Med.* 1995; 332:1529–1534.

Stone, A.B., Pearlstein, T.B., and Brown, W.K. Fluoxetine in the treatment of late luteal phase dysphoric disorder. *J. Clin. Psychiatry* 1991; 52:290–293.

Sunblad, C., Modigh, K., Andersch, B., et al. Clomipramine effectively reduces premenstrual irritability and dysphoria: a placebo-controlled trial. *Acta Psychiatr. Scand.* 1992; 85:39–47.

Wood, S.H., Mortola, J.F., Yuen-Fai, C., et al. Treatment of premenstrual syndrome with fluoxetine: a double-blind placebo-controlled crossover study. *Obstet. Gynecol.* 1992; 80:339–344.

Yonkers, K.A. Antidepressants in the treatment of premenstrual dysphoric disorder. *J. Clin. Psychiatry* 1997; 58(supplement 14): 4–13.

Yonkers, K.A., and Brown, W.A. Pharmacologic treatments for premenstrual dysphoric disorder. *Psychiatric Annals* 1996; 26:586–589.

Yonkers, K.A., Gullion, C., Williams, A., et al. Paroxetine as a treatment for premenstrual dysphoric disorder. *J. Clin. Psychopharmacol.* 1996; 16:3–8.

Yonkers, K.A., Halbreich, U., Freeman, E.W., et al. Sertraline in the treatment of premenstrual dysphoric disorder. *Psychopharmacol. Bull.* 1996; 32:41–46.

Young, S.A., Hurt, P.H., Benedek, D.M., and Howard, R.S. Treatment of premenstrual dysphoric disorder with sertraline during the luteal phase: a randomized, double-blind, placebo-controlled trial. *J. Clin. Psychiatry* 1998; 59:76–80.

Other Medical Conditions

Abbey, S.E., and Garfinkel, P.E. Neurasthenia and chronic fatigue syndrome. The role of culture in the making of a diagnosis. *Am. J. Psychiatry* 1991; 148:1638–1646.

Adly, C., Straumanis, J., and Chesson, A. Fluoxetine prophylaxis of migraine. *Headache* 1992; 32:101–104.

Althof, S.E., Levine, S.B., Corty, E.W., et al. A double-blind crossover trial of clomipramine for rapid ejaculation in 15 couples. *J. Clin. Psychiatry* 1995; 56:402–407.

Breitbart, W., and Holland, J.C. (eds.). *Psychiatric Aspects of Symptom Management in Cancer Patients.* American Psychiatric Press, Washington, DC, 1994.

Cannon, R., Quyyum, A.A., Mincemoyer, R., et al. Imipramine in patients with chest pain despite normal coronary angiograms. *N. Engl. J. Med.* 1994; 330:1411–1417.

Clouse, R.E. Antidepressants for functional gastrointestinal syndromes. *Dig. Dis. Sci.* 1994; 39:2352–2363.

Couch, J.R., and Hassanein, R.S. Amitriptyline in migraine prophylaxis. *Arch. Neurol.* 1979; 36:695–699.

Couch, J.R., Ziegler, D.K., and Hassanein, R.S. Amitriptyline in the prophylaxis of migraine. *Neurology* 1976; 26:121–127.

Diamond, S., and Baltes, B.J. Chronic tension headaches treated with amitriptyline: a double-blind study. *Headache* 1971; 11:110–116.

Dwight, M.M., Arnold, L.M., O'Brien, H., et al. An open clinical trial of venlafaxine treatment of fibromyalgia. *Psychosomatics* 1998; 39:14–17.

Elliot, A.J., Uldall, K.K., Bergam, K., et al. Randomized, placebo-controlled trial of paroxetine versus imipramine in depressed HIV-positive outpatients. *Am. J. Psychiatry* 1998; 155:367–372.

Evans, D.L., Staab, J.P., Petitto, J.M., et al. Depression in the medical setting: biopsychological interactions and treatment considerations. *J. Clin. Psychiatry* 1999; 60:40–56.

Feinmann, C. Pain relief by antidepressants: possible modes of action. *Pain* 1985; 23:1–8.

France, R.D. The future of antidepressants: treatment of pain. *Psychopathology* 1987; 20(supplement 1):99–113.

France, R.D., Haupt, J.L., and Ellinwood, E.H. Therapeutic effects of antidepressants in chronic pain. *Gen. Hosp. Psychiatry* 1984; 6:55–63.

Goodnick, P.J., and Sandoval, R. Psychotropic treatment of chronic fatigue syndrome and related disorders. *J. Clin. Psychiatry* 1993; 54:13–20.

Hameroff, S.R., Cork, R.C., Scherer, K., et al. Doxepin effects on chronic pain, depression, and plasma opioids. *J. Clin. Psychiatry* 1982; 43:22–26.

Hameroff, S.R., Weiss, J.L., Lerman, J.C., et al. Doxepin's effects on chronic pain and depression: a controlled study. *J. Clin. Psychiatry* 1984; 45:3(sec. 2):47–52.

Hendler, N. The anatomy and psychopharmacology of chronic pain. *J. Clin. Psychiatry* 1982; 43:15–20.

Hudson, J.I., Hudson, M.S., Pliner, L.F., et al. Fibromyalgia and major affective disorder: a controlled phenomenology and family history study. *Am. J. Psychiatry* 1985; 142:441–446.

Katon, W.J., and Walker, E.A. Medically unexplained symptoms in primary care. *J. Clin. Psychiatry* 1998; 59(supplement 20):15–21.

Krishnan, R.R., and France, R.D. Antidepressants in chronic pain syndromes. *Am. Fam. Physician* 1989; 39:233–237.

Kvinesdal, B., Molin, J., Froland, A., et al. Imipramine treatment of painful diabetic neuropathy. *JAMA* 1984; 251:1727–1730.

Lance, J.W., and Curran, D.A. Treatment of chronic tension headache. *Lancet* 1964; 1:1236–1239.

Lee, H.S., Song, D.H., Kim, C.H., Choi, H.K. An open clinical trial of fluoxetine in the treatment of premature ejaculation. *J. Clin. Psychopharmacol.* 1996; 16:379–382.

Mahloudji, M. Prevention of migraine. *Br. Med. J.* 1969; 1:182–183.

Masand, P.S., Kaplan, D.S., Gupta, S., and Bhandary, A.N. Major depression and irritable bowel syndrome (IBS): is there a relationship? *J. Clin. Psychiatry* 1995; 56:363–365.

———. Irritable bowel syndrome and dysthymia: is there a relationship? *Psychosomatics* 1997; 38:63–69.

Max, M.B., Lynch, S.A., Muir, J., et al. Effects of desipramine, amitriptyline, and fluoxetine on pain in diabetic neuropathy. *N. Engl. J. Med.* 1992; 326:1250–1256.

Mendels, J., Camera, A., Sikes, C. Sertraline treatment for premature ejaculation. *J. Clin. Psychopharmacol.* 1995; 15:341–346.

Nowell, P.D., Reynolds, C.F., Buysse, D.J., et al. Paroxetine in the treatment of primary insomnia: preliminary clinical and electroencephalogram sleep data. *J. Clin. Psychiatry* 1999; 60:89–95.

Noyes, R., Cook, B., Garvey, M., et al. Reduction of gastrointestinal symptoms following treatment for panic disorder. *Psychosomatics* 1990; 31:75–79.

Okasha, A., Ghaleb, H.A., and Sedek, A. A double-blind trial for the clinical management of psychogenic headache. *Br. J. Psychiatry* 1973; 122:181–183.

Orsulak, P.J., and Waller, D. Antidepressant drugs: additional clinical uses. *J. Fam. Pract.* 1989; 28:209–216.

Peatfield, R.C., Fozard, J.R., and Rose, F.C. Drug treatment of migraine. In Rose, F.C. (ed.). *Handbook of Clinical Neurology.* Elsevier Publishers, New York, 1986.

Rabkin, J.G., Wagner, G.J., and Rabkin, R. Fluoxetine treatment of depression in patients with HIV and AIDS: a randomized, placebo-controlled trial. *Am. J. Psychiatry* 1999; 156:101–107.

Sakal, F., and Meyer, J.S. Abnormal cerebrovascular reactivity in patients with migraine and cluster headache. *Headache* 1979; 19:257–266.

Segraves, R.T. Effects of psychotropic drugs on human erection and ejaculation. *Arch. Gen. Psychiatry* 1989; 46:275–284.

Sindrup, A.S.H., Gram, L.F., Brosen, K., et al. The selective serotonin reuptake inhibitor paroxetine is effective in the treatment of diabetic neuropathy symptoms. *Pain* 1990; 42:135–144.

Spiegel, K., Calb, R., and Pasternak, G.W. Analgesic activity of tricyclic antidepressants. *Ann. Neurol.* 1983; 13:462–465.

Stein, D., Peri, T., Edelstein, E., et al. The efficacy of amitriptyline and acetaminophen in the management of acute low back pain. *Psychosomatics* 1996; 37:63–70.

Stewart, J.T., and Shin, K.J. Paroxetine treatment of sexual disinhibition in dementia. *Am. J. Psychiatry* 1997; 154:1474.

Stoudemire, A., and Fogel, B.S. (eds.). *Psychiatric Care of the Medical Patient.* Oxford University Press, New York, 1993.

Tollefson, G.D., Tollefson, L., and Pederson, M. Comorbid irritable bowel syndrome in patients with generalized anxiety disorder and major depression. *Ann. Clin. Psychiatry* 1991; 3:215–222.

Waldinger, M.D., Hengeveld, M.W., and Zwinderman, A.H. Paroxetine treatment of premature ejaculation: a double-blind, randomized, placebo-controlled study. *Am. J. Psychiatry* 1994; 151:1377–1379.

Walker, E.A., Roy-Byrne, P.P., Katon, W.J., et al. Psychiatric illness and irritable bowel syndrome: a comparison with inflammatory bowel disease. *Am. J. Psychiatry* 1990; 147:1656–1661.

Walsh, T.D. Antidepressants and chronic pain. *Clin. Neuropharmacol.* 1983; 6:271–295.

Ward, N.G., Bloom, V.L., and Friedel, R.O. The effectiveness of tricyclic antidepressants in the treatment of coexisting pain and depression. *Pain* 1979; 7:331–341.

Ware, N.C., and Kleinman, A. Depression in neurasthenia and chronic fatigue syndrome. *Psychiatric Annals* 1992; 22:202–208.

Watson, C.P., Evans, R.J., Reed, K., et al. Amitriptyline versus placebo in postherpetic neuralgia. *Neurology* 1982; 36:671–673.

Watson, C.P.N. Therapeutic window for amitriptyline analgesia. *Can. Med. Assoc. J.* 1984; 130:105.

Placebo

Stewart, J.W., Quitkin, F.M., McGrath, P.J., et al. Use of pattern analysis to predict differential relapse of remitted patients with major depression during one year of treatment with fluoxetine or placebo. *Arch. Gen. Psychiatry* 1998; 55:334–343.

Straus, J.L., and Cavanaugh, S.V. Placebo effects: issues for clinical practice in psychiatry and medicine. *Psychosomatics* 1996; 37:315–326.

Suicidality/Violence

Bruun, R.D., Budman, C.L. Paroxetine treatment of episodic rages associated with Tourette's disorder. *J. Clin. Psychiatry* 1998; 59:581–584.

Burton, T.M. Anti-depression drug of Eli Lilly loses sales after attack by sect. Scientologists claim Prozac induces murder or suicide, though evidence is scant. *Wall Street Journal,* April 19, 1991.

————. Panel finds no credible evidence to tie Prozac to suicides and violent behavior. *Wall Street Journal,* September 23, 1991.

Coccaro, E.F., and Kavoussi, R.J. Fluoxetine and impulse aggressive behavior in personality-disordered subjects. *Arch. Gen. Psychiatry* 1997; 54:1081–1088.

Fava, M. Psychopharmacologic treatment of pathologic aggression. *Psychiatr. Clin. North Am.* 1997; 20:427–451.

Fava, M., and Rosenbaum, J.F. Suicidality and fluoxetine: is there a relationship? *J. Clin. Psychiatry* 1991; 52:108–111.

FDA Talk Paper: FDA denies Scientology petition against Prozac. U.S. Department of Health and Human Services, Rockville, MD, August 1, 1991.

Leon, A.C., Keller, M.B., Warshaw, M.G., et al. Prospective study of fluoxetine treatment and suicidal behavior in affectively ill subjects. *Am. J. Psychiatry* 1999; 156:195–201.

Moses, J. Suits over Prozac likely to continue although no link was found to violence. *Wall Street Journal,* September 24, 1991.

Muller-Oerlinghausen, B., and Berghofer, A. Antidepressants and suicidal risk. *J. Clin. Psychiatry* 1999; 60(supplement 2):95–99.

Rubey, R.N., Johnson, M.R., Emmanuel, N., and Lydiard, R.B. Fluoxetine in the treatment of anger: an open trial. *J. Clin. Psychiatry* 1996; 57:398–401.

Salzman, C., Wolfson, A.N., Schatzberg, A., et al. Effect of fluoxetine on anger in symptomatic volunteers with borderline personality disorder. *J. Clin. Psychopharmacol.* 1995; 15:23–29.

Teicher, M.H., Glod, C., and Cole, J.O. Emergence of intense suicidal preoccupation during fluoxetine treatment. *Am. J. Psychiatry* 1990; 147:207–210.

Tollefson, G.D., Fawcett, J., Winokur, G., et al. Evaluation of suicidality during pharmacologic treatment of mood and non-mood disorders. *Ann. Clin. Psychiatry* 1993; 5:209–214.

Verkes, R.J., Van der Mast, R.C., Hengeveld, M.W., et al. Reduction by paroxetine of suicidal behavior in patients with repeated suicide attempts but not major depression. *Am. J. Psychiatry* 1998; 155:543–547.

Warshaw, M.G., and Keller, M.B. The relationship between fluoxetine use and suicidal behavior in 654 subjects with anxiety disorder. *J. Clin. Psychiatry* 1996; 57:158–166.

2

Medical Factors

Brown, T.M., and Stoudemire, A. *Psychiatric Side Effects of Prescription and Over-the-Counter Medications.* American Psychiatric Press, Washington, DC, 1998.

Cameron, O.G. (ed.). *Presentations of Depression: Depression in Medical and Other Psychiatric Disorders.* John Wiley & Sons, New York, 1987.

Cummings, J.L. Depression in neurological diseases. *Psychiatric Annals* 1994; 24:525–531.

———. Dementia and depression: an evolving enigma. *J. Neuropsychiatry Clin. Neurosci.* 1989; 1:236–242.

Eisendraph, S.J., and Sweeney, M.A. Toxic neuropsychiatric effects of digoxin at therapeutic serum concentrations. *Am. J. Psychiatry* 1987; 144:506–507.

Gadde, K.M., and Krishnan, K.R.K. Endocrine factors in depression. *Psychiatric Annals* 1994; 24:521–524.

Gelenberg, A.J. Depression, depressants, and antidepressants. *Arch. Intern. Med.* 1990; 150:22–45.

Glassman, A.H. Cardiovascular effects of antidepressant drugs: updated. *J. Clin. Psychiatry* 1998; 59(supplement 15):13–18.

Glassman, A.H., Rodriguez, A.I., and Shapiro, P.A. The use of antidepressant drugs in patients with heart disease. *J. Clin. Psychiatry* 1998; 59(supplement 10):16–21.

Goodnick, P.J., Henry, J.H., and Buci, V.M. Treatment of depression in patients with diabetes mellitus. *J. Clin. Psychiatry* 1995; 56:128–136.

Hall, R.C., Gardner, E.R., Popkin, M.K., et al. Unrecognized physical illness prompting psychiatric admission: a prospective study. *Am. J. Psychiatry* 1981; 130:629–635.

Holdiness, M.R. Neurological manifestations and toxicities of the antituberculosis drugs: a review. *Med. Toxicol.* 1987; 2:33–51.

Koranyi, E.K. Somatic illness in psychiatric patients. *Psychosomatics* 1980; 21:887–891.

Kurtz, S., Ashkenazi, I., and Melamed, S. Major depressive episode secondary to antiglaucoma drugs. *Am. J. Psychiatry* 1993; 150:524–525.

Lechleitner, M., Hoppichler, F., Konwalinka, G., et al. Depressive symptoms in hypercholesterolemia treated with pravastatin. *Lancet* 1992; 340:910.

Lewis, D.A., and Smith, R.E. Steroid-induced psychiatric syndromes. *J. Affect. Disord.* 1983; 5:319–332.

Long, T.D., and Kathol, R.G. Critical review of data supporting affective disorder caused by nonpsychotropic medication. *Ann. Clin. Psychiatry* 1993; 5:259–270.

Malone, D.A., and Dimeff, R.J. Use of fluoxetine in depression associated with anabolic steroid withdrawal: a case series. *J. Clin. Psychiatry* 1992; 53:130–132.

McDonald, E.M., Mann, A.H., and Thomas, H.C. Interferons as mediators of psychiatric morbidity: an investigation in a trial of recombinant alpha-interferon in hepatitis-B carriers. *Lancet* 1987; 11:1175–1178.

Metzger, E.D., and Friedman, R.S. Treatment-related depression. *Psychiatric Annals* 1994; 24:540–551.

Morrison, J. *When Psychological Problems Mask Medical Disorders: A Guide for Psychotherapists.* Guilford Publications, New York, 1997.

Pies, R.W. Medical "mimics" of depression. *Psychiatric Annals* 1994; 24:519–520.

Pope, H.G., and Katz, D.L. Psychiatric and medical effects of anabolic-androgenic steroid use. *Arch. Gen. Psychiatry* 1994; 51:375–382.

Robertson, M.M., Trimble, M.R., and Townsend, H.R. Phenomenology of depression in epilepsy. *Epilepsia* 1987; 28:364–372.

Roose, S.P., Glassman, A.H., et al. Tricyclic antidepressants in depressed patients with cardiac conduction disease. *Arch. Gen. Psychiatry* 1987; 44:273–275.

Rundell, J.R., and Wise, M.C. (eds.). *Textbook of Consultation-Liaison Psychiatry.* American Psychiatric Press, Washington, DC, 1996.

Russell, G.R., and Wise, M.G. Causes of organic mood disorder. *J. Neuropsychiatry Clin. Neurosci.* 1989; 1:398–400.

Stoudemire, A., Brown, J.T., Harris, R.T., et al. Propranolol and depression: a re-evaluation based on a pilot clinical trial. *Psychiatr. Med.* 1984; 2:211–218.

Townes, B.D., Bashein, G., Horbein, T.F., et al. Neurobehavioral outcomes in cardiac operations. *J. Thorac. Cardiovasc. Surg.* 1989; 98:774–782.

Wamboldt, F.S., Jefferson, J.W., and Wamboldt, M.Z. Digitalis intoxication misdiagnosed as depression by primary care physicians. *Am. J. Psychiatry* 1986; 143:219–221.

Winokur, G., Black, D.W., and Nasarallah, H. Depressions secondary to other psychiatric disorders and medical illnesses. *Am. J. Psychiatry* 1988; 145:223–237.

Yudofski, S.C. Beta-blockers and depression: the clinician's dilemma. *JAMA* 1992; 267:1826–1827.

Triggering Mania

Altshuler, L.L., Post, R.M., Levrich, G.S., et al. Antidepressant-induced mania and cycle acceleration: a controversy revisited. *Am. J. Psychiatry* 1995; 152:1130–1138.

Angst, J. Switch from depression to mania, or from mania to depression: role of psychotropic drugs. *Psychopharmacol. Bull.* 1987; 23:66–67.

Bauer, M.S., Callahan, A.M., Jampala, C., et al. Clinical practice guidelines for bipolar disorder from the Department of Veteran Affairs. *J. Clin. Psychiatry* 1999; 60:9–21.

Boerlin, H.L., Gitlin, M.J., Zoellner, L.A., and Hammen C. Bipolar depression and antidepressant-induced mania: a naturalistic study. *J. Clin. Psychiatry* 1998; 59:374–379.

Frances, A.J., Kahn, D.A., Carpenter, D., et al. The expert consensus guidelines for treating depression in bipolar disorder. *J. Clin. Psychiatry* 1998; 59(supplement 4):73–79.

Kupfer, D.J., Carpenter, L.L., and Frank, E. Possible role of antidepressants in precipitating mania and hypomania in recurrent depression. *Am. J. Psychiatry* 1988; 145:804–808.

Peet, M. Induction of mania with selective serotonin reuptake inhibitors and tricyclic antidepressants. *Br. J. Psychiatry* 1994; 164:549–550.

Potter, W.Z. Bipolar disorder: specific treatments. *J. Clin. Psychiatry* 1998; 59(supplement 18):30–36.

Simpson, H.B., Hurowitz, G.I., and Liebowitz, M.R. General principles in the pharmacotherapy of antidepressant-induced rapid cycling: a case series. *J. Clin. Psychopharmacol.* 1997; 17:460–466.

Solomon, R.L., Rich, C.L., and Darko, D.F. Antidepressant treatment and the occurrence of mania in bipolar patients admitted for depression. *J. Affect. Disord.* 1990; 18:253–257.

Stoll, A.L., Mayer, P.V., Kolbrenner, M., et al. Antidepressant-associated mania: a controlled comparison with spontaneous mania. *Am. J. Psychiatry* 1994; 151:1642–1645.

Wehr, T.A., and Goodwin, F.K. Rapid cycling in manic-depressives induced by tricyclic antidepressants. *Arch. Gen. Psychiatry* 1979; 36:555–559.

————. Do antidepressants cause mania? *Psychopharmacol. Bull.* 1987; 23:61–65.

————. Can antidepressants cause mania and worsen the course of affective illness? *Am. J. Psychiatry* 1987; 144:1403–1411.

Wehr, T.A., Sack, D.A., Rosenthal, N.E., and Cowdry, R.W. Rapid cycling affective disorder: contributing factors and treatment responses in 51 patients. *Am. J. Psychiatry* 1988; 145:179–184.

Genetics

Biederman, J. Faraone, S.V., Keenan, K., et al. Further evidence of family-genetic risk factors in attention deficit hyperactivity disorder: patters of comorbidity in probands and relatives in psychiatrically and pediatrically referred samples. *Arch. Gen. Psychiatry* 1992; 49:728–738.

Cadoret, R.J., Winokur, G., Langbehn, D., et al. Depression spectrum disease, I: the role of gene-environment interaction. *Am. J. Psychiatry* 1996; 153:892–899.

Kassett, J.A., Gershon, E.S., Maxwell, M.E., et al. Psychiatric disorders in the first-degree relatives of probands with bulimia nervosa. *Am. J. Psychiatry* 1989; 146:1468–1471.

Kendler, K.S., Heath, A.C., Martin, N.G., and Eaves, L.J. Symptoms of anxiety and depression in a volunteer twin population: the etiologic role of genetic and environmental factors. *Arch. Gen. Psychiatry* 1986; 43:213–221.

Kendler, K.S., Kessler, R.C., Walters, E.E., MacLean, C., et al. Stressful life events, genetic liability, and onset of an episode of major depression in women. *Am. J. Psychiatry* 1995; 152:833–842.

Kendler, K.S., MacLean, C.J., Neale, M.C., et al. The genetic epidemiology of bulimia nervosa. *Am. J. Psychiatry* 1991; 148:1627–1637.

Kendler, K.S., Neale, M.C., Kessler, R.C., et al. A population-based twin study of major depression in women: the impact of varying definitions of illness. *Arch. Gen. Psychiatry* 1992; 49:257–266.

Kendler, K.S., Neale, M.C., Kessler, R.C., et al. Generalized anxiety disorder in women: a population-based twin study. *Arch. Gen. Psychiatry* 1992; 49:267–272.

Kendler, K.S., Neale, M.C., Kessler, R.C., et al. The genetic epidemiology of phobias in women: the interrelationship of agoraphobia, social phobia, situational phobia, and simple phobia. *Arch. Gen. Psychiatry* 1992; 49:273–281.

Kendler, K.S., and Prescott, C.A. A population-based twin study of lifetime major depression in men and women. *Arch. Gen. Psychiatry* 1999; 56:39–44.

Kendler, K.S., Walters, E.E., Neale, M.C., et al. The structure of the genetic environmental factors for six major psychiatric disorders in women. *Arch. Gen. Psychiatry* 1995; 52:374–383.

Madden, P.A.F., Heath, A.C., Rosenthal, N.E., and Martin, N.G. Seasonal changes in mood and behavior: the role of genetic factors. *Arch. Gen. Psychiatry* 1996; 53:47–55.

Merikangas, K.R., Leckman, J.F., Prusoff, B.A., et al. Familial transmission of depression and alcoholism. *Arch. Gen. Psychiatry* 1985; 42:367–372.

Pauls, D.L., Brook, J.P. II, Goodman, W., et al. A family study of obsessive-compulsive disorder. *Am. J. Psychiatry* 1995; 152:76–84.

Rasmussen, S.A., and Tsuang, M.T. Clinical characteristics and family history in DSM-III obsessive-compulsive disorder. *Am. J. Psychiatry* 1986; 143:317–322.

Torgerson, S. Genetic factors in anxiety disorder. *Arch. Gen. Psychiatry* 1983; 40:1085–1087.

True, W.R., Rice, J., Eisen, S.A., et al. A twin study of genetic and environmental contribution to liability for posttraumatic stress symptoms. *Arch. Gen. Psychiatry* 1993; 50:257–264.

Tsuang, M.T., and Faraone, S.V. *The Genetics of Mood Disorders*. Johns Hopkins University Press, Baltimore, 1990.

Tsuang, M.T., and VanderMey, R. *Genes and the Mind: Inheritance of Mental Illness*. Oxford University Press, New York, 1980.

Walters, E.E., and Kendler, K.S. Anorexia nervosa, and anorexic-like syndromes in a population-based female twin sample. *Am. J. Psychiatry* 1995; 152:64–71.

Depression with Psychotic Features

Chan, C.H., Janicak, P.G., Davis, J.M., et al. Response of psychotic and nonpsychotic depressed patients to tricyclic antidepressants. *J. Clin. Psychiatry* 1987; 48:197–200.

Coryell, W. The treatment of psychotic depression. *J. Clin. Psychiatry* 1998; 59(supplement 1):22–27.

Coryell, W., Keller, M., Lavori, P., et al. Affective syndromes, psychotic features, and prognosis: 1. Depression. *Arch. Gen. Psychiatry* 1990; 47:651–657.

Dubovsky, S.L., and Thomas, M. Psychotic depression: advances in conceptualization and treatment. *Hosp. Community Psychiatry* 1992; 43:1189–1198.

Frances, A., Brown, R.P., Kocsis, J.H., et al. Psychotic depression: a separate entity? *Am. J. Psychiatry* 1981; 138:831–833.

Janicak, P.G., Pandey, G.N., Davis, J.M., et al. Response of psychotic and nonpsychotic depression to phenelzine. *Am. J. Psychiatry* 1988; 145:93–95.

Kocsis, J.H., Croughan, J.L., Katz, M.M., et al. Response to treatment with antidepressants of patients with severe or moderate nonpsychotic depression and of patients with psychotic depression. *Am. J. Psychiatry* 1990; 147:621–624.

Mazure, C.M., Nelson, J.C., Jarlow, P.I., et al. The relationship between blood perphenazine levels, early resolution of psychotic symptoms, and side effects. *J. Clin. Psychiatry* 1990; 51:330–334.

Mulsant, B.H., Hasket, R.F., Prudic, J., et al. Low use of neuroleptic drugs in the treatment of psychotic major depression. *Am. J. Psychiatry* 1997; 154:559–561.

Nelson, J.C., and Bowers, M.B. Delusional versus unipolar depression: description and drug response. *Arch. Gen. Psychiatry* 1978; 35:1321–1328.

Nelson, W.H., Khan, A., and Orr, W.W. Delusional depression: phenomenology, neuroendocrine function, and tricyclic antidepressant response. *J. Affect. Disord.* 1984; 6:297–306.

Quitkin, F., Rifkin, A., and Klein, D.F. Imipramine response in deluded depressive patients. *Am. J. Psychiatry* 1978; 135:806–811.

Rothschild, A.J., Bates, K.S., Boehringer, K.L., and Syed, A. Olanzapine response in psychotic depression. *J. Clin. Psychiatry* 1999; 60:116–118.

Rothschild, A.J., Samson, J.A., Besette, M.P., and Carter-Campbell, J.T. Efficacy of combination fluoxetine and perphenazine in the treatment of psychotic depression. *J. Clin. Psychiatry* 1993; 54:338–342.

Schatzberg, A.F., and Rothschild, A.J. Psychotic (delusional) major depression: should it be included as a distinct syndrome in DSM-IV? *Am. J. Psychiatry* 1992; 149:733–745.

Spiker, D.G., Perel, J.M., Hanin, I., et al. The pharmacological treatment of delusional depression: Part II. *J. Clin. Psychopharmacol.* 1984; 4:311–315.

Alcohol, Caffeine, and Recreational Drugs

American Psychiatric Association. Practice guideline for treatment of patients with substance use disorders: alcohol, cocaine, opioids. *Am. J. Psychiatry* 1995; 152(11, supplement):5–59.

Anthenelli, R.M. The initial evaluation of the dual diagnosis patient. *Psychiatric Annals* 1994; 24:407–411.

Anthenelli, R.M., and Schuckit, M.A. Affective and anxiety disorders and alcohol and drug dependency: diagnosis and treatment. *J. Addictive Diseases* 1993; 12:73–87.

Behar, D., and Winokur, G. Depression in the abstinent alcoholic. *Am. J. Psychiatry* 1984; 141:1106–1107.

Brady, K.T., and Roberts, J.M. The pharmacotherapy of dual diagnosis. *Psychiatric Annals* 1995; 25:344–352.

Brown, S.A., Inaba, R.K., Gillin, J.C., et al. Alcoholism and affective disorder: clinical course of depressive symptoms. *Am. J. Psychiatry* 1995; 152:45–52.

Castenada, R., Sussman, N., Westreich, L., et al. A review of the effects of moderate alcohol intake on the treatment of anxiety and mood disorders. *J. Clin. Psychiatry* 1996; 57:207–212.

Charney, D.S., Heninger, G.R., and Jatlow, P.I. Increased anxiogenic effects of caffeine in panic disorders. *Arch. Gen. Psychiatry* 1985; 42:233–243.

Cornelius, J.R., Salloum, I.M., Ehler, J.G., et al. Fluoxetine in depressed alcoholics: a double-blind, placebo-controlled trial. *Arch. Gen. Psychiatry* 1997; 54:700–705.

Dackis, C.A., Gold, M.S., Pottash, A.L., and Sweeny, D.R. Evaluating depression in alcoholics. *Psychiatry Res.* 1986; 17:105–109.

Galanter, M., Egelko, S., DeLeon, G., et al. Crack/cocaine abusers in the general hospital: assessment and initiation of care. *Am. J. Psychiatry* 1992; 149:810–815.

Galanter, M., and Kleber, H.D. (eds.). *The American Psychiatric Press Textbook of Substance Abuse Treatment, Second Edition.* American Psychiatric Press, Washington, DC, 1999.

Greden, J.F. Anxiety or caffeinism: a diagnostic dilemma. *Am. J. Psychiatry* 1974; 131:1089–1092.

Greden, J.F., Fontaine, P., Lubetsky, M., and Chamberlin, K. Anxiety and depression associated with caffeinism among psychiatric in-patients. *Am. J. Psychiatry* 1978; 135:963–966.

Greenfield, S.F., Weiss, R.D., Muenz, L.R., et al. The effect of de-pression on return to drinking: a prospective study. *Arch. Gen. Psychiatry* 1998; 55:259–265.

Hughes, J.R., Oliveto, A.H., and Helzer, J.E. Should caffeine abuse, dependence, or withdrawal be added to DSM-IV and ICD-10? *Am. J. Psychiatry* 1992; 149:33–40.

Longo, L.P. Non-benzodiazepine pharmacotherapy of anxiety and panic in substance abusing patients. *Psychiatric Annals* 1998; 28:142–153.

Longo, L.P., and Johnson, B. Treatment of insomnia in substance abusing patients. *Psychiatric Annals* 1998; 28:154–159.

Mason, B.J., Kocsis, J.H., Ritvo, E.C., and Cutler, R.B. A double-blind, placebo-controlled trial of desipramine for primary alcohol dependence stratified on the presence or absence of major depres-sion. *JAMA* 1996; 275:761–767.

McGrath, P.J., Nunes, E.V., Stewart, J.W., et al. Imipramine treat-ment of alcoholics with primary depression: a placebo-controlled clinical trial. *Arch. Gen. Psychiatry* 1996; 53:232–241.

Minkoff, K., and Drake, R.E. (eds.). *Dual Diagnosis of Major Mental Illness and Substance Disorder*. Jossey-Bass, San Francisco, 1991.

Nunes, E.V., McGrath, P.J., Quitkin, F.M., et al. Imipramine treat-ment of alcoholism with co-morbid depression. *Am. J. Psychiatry* 1993; 150:963–965.

Pope, H.G., and Yurgelun-Todd, D. The residual cognitive effects of heavy marijuana use in college students. *JAMA* 1996; 275:521–524.

Regier, D.A., Farmer, M.E., Rae, D.S., et al. Comorbidity of mental disorders with alcohol and other drug abuse. *JAMA* 1990; 264:2511–2518.

Renner, J.A., and Ciraulo, D.A. Substance abuse and depression. *Psy-chiatric Annals* 1994; 24:532–539.

Rounsaville, B.J., Anton, S.F., Carroll, K., et al. Psychiatric diagnosis of treatment-seeking cocaine abusers. *Arch. Gen. Psychiatry* 1991; 48:43–50.

Schnoll, S.H., and Daghestani, A.N. Treatment of marijuana abuse. *Psychiatric Annals* 1986; 16:249–254.

Schuckit, M.A. *Drug and Alcohol Abuse: A Clinical Guide to Diagnosis and Treatment, Third Edition*. Plenum Press, New York, 1989.

———. Alcoholic patients with secondary depression. *Am. J. Psychiatry* 1983; 140:711–714.

Schuckit, M.A., Tipp, J.E., Bergman, M., et al. Comparison of induced and independent major depressive disorders in 2,945 alcoholics. *Am. J. Psychiatry* 1997; 154:948–957.

Stoll, A.L., Cole, J.O., and Lucas, S.E. A case of mania as a result of fluoxetine-marijuana interaction. *J. Clin. Psychiatry* 1991; 52:280–281.

Weiss, R.D., and Mirin, S.M. The dual diagnosis alcoholic: evaluation and treatment. *Psychiatric Annals* 1989; 19:261–265.

Weiss, R.D., Mirin, S.M., Michael, J.L., and Sollogub, A.C. Psychopathology in chronic cocaine abusers. *Am. J. Drug Alcohol Abuse* 1986; 12:17–29.

Weissman, M.M., and Meyers, J.K. Clinical depression in alcoholism. *Am. J. Psychiatry* 1980; 137:372–373.

Wilens, T.E., Biederman, J., and Spencer, T.J. Case study: adverse effects of smoking marijuana while receiving tricyclic antidepressants. *J. Am. Acad. Child Adolesc. Psychiatry* 1997; 36:45–48.

Antidepressant Choice

Barbey, J.T., and Roose, S.P. SSRI safety in overdose. *J. Clin. Psychiatry* 1998; 59(supplement 15):42–48.

Efremova, I., and Asnis, G. Antidepressants in depressed patients with irritable bowel syndrome. *Am. J. Psychiatry* 1998; 155:1627–1628.

Liebowitz, M.R., Quitkin, F.M., McGrath, P.J., et al. Antidepressant specificity in atypical depression. *Arch. Gen. Psychiatry* 1988; 45:129–137.

Nelson, J.C. Treatment in antidepressant nonresponders: augmentation or switch? *J. Clin. Psychiatry* 1998; 59(supplement 15):35–41.

Nierenberg, A.A. Treatment choice after one antidepressant fails: a survey of northeastern psychiatrists. *J. Clin. Psychiatry* 1991; 52:383–385.

Nobler, M.S., and Roose, S.P. Differential response to antidepressants in melancholic and severe depression. *Psychiatric Annals* 1998; 28:84–88.

Olfson, M., Maarcus, S.C., Pincus, H.A., et al. Antidepressant prescribing practices of outpatient psychiatrists. *Arch. Gen. Psychiatry* 1998; 55:310–316.

Perry, P.J. Pharmacotherapy for major depression with melancholic features: relative efficacy of tricyclic versus selective serotonin reuptake inhibitor antidepressants. *J. Affect. Disord.* 1996; 39:1–6.

Preskorn, S.H. Antidepressant drug selection: criteria and options. *J. Clin. Psychiatry* 1994; 55(supplement A):6–22.

Quitkin, F.M., McGrath, P.J., Stewart, J.W., et al. Chronological milestones to guide drug change: when should clinicians switch antidepressants. *Arch. Gen. Psychiatry* 1996; 53:783–792.

Stahl, S.M. Selecting an antidepressant by using mechanism of action to enhance efficacy and avoid side effects. *J. Clin. Psychiatry* 1998; 59(supplement 18):23–29.

Steffens, D.C., and Krishnan, K.R.R. Using a decision model to compare SSRIs and TCAs. *Primary Psychiatry* 1998; 5:79–84.

Generic Medication

Cohen, L.J. Commonly asked questions about trade name vs. generic pharmaceutical products. *J. Clin. Psychiatry* 1997; 4(monograph 15):2–6.

Lamy, P.P. Generic equivalents: issues and concerns. *J. Clin. Pharmacol.* 1986; 26:309–316.

Nightengale, S.C., and Morrison, J.C. Generic drugs and the prescribing physician. *JAMA* 1987; 258:1200–1204.

Rosenbaum, J.F., Charney, D.S., Fawcett, J.A., et al. Generic drugs: a roundtable discussion. *J. Clin. Psychiatry* 1989; 7(monograph 1).

Blood Levels

American Psychiatric Association Task Force. Tricyclic antidepressants—blood level measurements and clinical outcome: an APA Task Force report. *Am. J. Psychiatry* 1985; 142:155–162.

Amsterdam, J., Brunswick, D., and Mendels, J. The clinical application of tricyclic antidepressant pharmacokinetics and plasma levels. *Am. J. Psychiatry* 1980; 137:653–662.

Amsterdam, J., Fawcett, J., Quitkin, F.M., et al. Fluoxetine and norfluoxetine plasma concentrations in major depression: a multicenter study. *Am. J. Psychiatry* 1997; 154:963–969.

Asberg, M., Cronholm, B., Sjoqvist, F., and Tuck, D. Relationship between plasma level and therapeutic effect of nortriptyline. *Br. Med. J.* 1971; 3:331–334.

Breyer-Pfaff, U., Giedke, H., Gaertner, H.J., and Nill, K. Validation of a therapeutic plasma level range in amitriptyline treatment of depression. *J. Clin. Psychopharmacol.* 1989; 9:116–121.

Brunswick, D.J., Amsterdam, J.D., Potter, L., et al. Relationship between tricyclic antidepressant plasma levels and clinical response in patients treated with desipramine or doxepin. *Acta Psychiatr. Scand.* 1983; 67:371–377.

Fink, M., Glassman, A.H., and Davis, J.M. Question the experts. *J. Clin. Psychopharmacol.* 1993; 13:296–299.

Glassman, A.H., Perel, J.M., Shostak, M., et al. Clinical implications of imipramine plasma levels for depressive illness. *Arch. Gen. Psychiatry* 1977; 34:197–204.

Jerling, M. Dosing of antidepressants—the unknown art. *J. Clin. Psychopharmacol.* 1995; 15:435–439.

Nelson, J.C., Jatlow, P., and Mazure, C. Desipramine plasma concentration and response in elderly melancholic patients. *J. Clin. Psychopharmacol.* 1985; 5:217–220.

Orsulak, P.J. Therapeutic monitoring of antidepressant drugs. Current methodology and applications. *J. Clin. Psychiatry* 1986; 47(supplement 10):39–50.

Perry, P.J., Zeilmann, C., and Arndt S. Tricyclic antidepressant concentrations in plasma: an estimate of their sensitivity and specificity as a predictor of response. *J. Clin. Psychopharmacol.* 1994; 14:230–240.

Preskorn, S.H. Therapeutic drug monitoring with tricyclic antidepressants: a response. *J. Clin. Psychopharmacol.* 1994; 14:277–278.

Preskorn, S.H., Dorey, R.C., and Jerkevitch, G.S. Therapeutic drug monitoring of tricyclic antidepressants. *J. Clin. Psychiatry.* 1988; 34:822–828.

Preskorn, S.H., and Fast, G. Therapeutic drug monitoring for antidepressants: efficacy, safety, and cost effectiveness. *J. Clin. Psychiatry* 1991; 52:23–33.

Maintenance Medication

Altamura, A.C., and Percudani, M. The use of antidepressants for long-term treatment of recurrent depression: rationale, current methodologies, and future directions. *J. Clin. Psychiatry* 1993; 54(supplement 8):29–37.

Doogan, D.P., and Caillard, V. Sertraline in the prevention of depression. *Br. J. Psychiatry* 1992; 160:217–222.

Frank, E., Kupfer, D.J., Perel, J.M., et al. Three-year outcomes for maintenance therapies in recurrent depression. *Arch. Gen. Psychiatry* 1990; 47:1093–1099.

————. Comparison of full-dose versus half-dose pharmacotherapy in the maintenance treatment of recurrent depression. *J. Affect. Disord.* 1993; 27:139–145.

Frank, E., Prien, R.F., Jarrett, J.B., et al. Conceptualization and rationale for consensus definitions of terms in major depressive disorder: response, remission, recovery, relapse, and recurrence. *Arch. Gen. Psychiatry* 1991; 48:851–855.

Friedman, R.A., Mitchell, J., and Kocsis, J.H. Re-treatment of relapse following desipramine discontinuation in dysthymia. *Am. J. Psychiatry* 1995; 152:926–928.

Greden, J.F. Antidepressant maintenance medications: when to discontinue and how to stop? *J. Clin. Psychiatry* 1993; 54(supplement 8):39–45.

Harrison, W., Rabkin, J., Stewart, J.W. Phenelzine for chronic depression: a study of continuation treatment. *J. Clin. Psychiatry* 1986; 47:346–349.

Hirschfeld, R.M.A. The long-term nature of depression. *Psychiatric Annals* 1996; 26:313–314.

Keller, M.B., Kocsis, J.H., Thase, M.E., et al. Maintenance phase efficacy of sertraline for recurrent depression. *JAMA* 1998; 280:1665–1672.

Kocsis, J.H., Francis, A.J., Voss, C.B., et al. Imipramine treatment for chronic depression. *Arch. Gen. Psychiatry* 1988; 45:253–257.

Kocsis, J.H., Friedman, R.A., Markowitz, J.C., et al. Maintenance treatment for chronic depression. *Arch. Gen. Psychiatry* 1996; 53:769–774.

Kocsis, J.H., Sutton, B.M., Frances, A.J. Long-term follow-up of chronic depression treated with imipramine. *J. Clin. Psychiatry* 1991; 52:56–59.

Kupfer, D.J., Frank, E., Perel, J.M., et al. Five-year outcome for maintenance therapies in recurring depression. *Arch. Gen. Psychiatry* 1992; 49:769–773.

Melfi, C.A., Chawla, A.J., Croghan, T.W., et al. The effects of adherence to antidepressant treatment guidelines on relapse and recurrence of depression. *Arch. Gen. Psychiatry* 1998; 55:1128–1132.

Montgomery, S.A., Dufour, H., Brion, S., et al. The prophylactic efficacy of fluoxetine in unipolar depression. *Br. J. Psychiatry* 1988; 153(supplement 3):69–76.

Mundo, E., Bareggi, S.R., Pirola, R., et al. Long-term pharmacotherapy of obsessive-compulsive disorder: a double-blind controlled study. *J. Clin. Psychiatry* 1997; 17:4–10.

NIMH/NIH Consensus Development Panel. Mood disorders: pharmacologic prevention of recurrences. *Am. J. Psychiatry* 1985; 142:469–476.

Prien, R.F., Kupfer, D.J., Mansky, F.A., et al. Drug treatment in prevention of recurrences in unipolar and bipolar affective disorders: report of the NIMH Collaborative Study Group. *Arch. Gen. Psychiatry* 1984; 41:1096–1104.

Reimherr, F.W., Amsterdam, J.D., Quitkin, F.M., et al. Optimal length of continuation therapy in depression: a prospective assessment during long-term fluoxetine treatment. *Am. J. Psychiatry* 1998; 155:1247–1253.

Reynolds, C.F., Frank, E., Perel, J.M., et al. High relapse rate after discontinuation of adjunctive medication for elderly patients with recurrent major depression. *Am. J. Psychiatry* 1996; 153:1418–1422.

Schatzberg, A.F. Course of depression in adults: treatment options. *Psychiatric Annals* 1996; 26:336–341.

Stewart, J.W., Tricamo, E., McGrath, P.J., and Quitkin, F.M. Prophylactic efficacy of phenelzine and imipramine in chronic atypical depression: likelihood of recurrence on discontinuation after 6 months' remission. *Am. J. Psychiatry* 1997; 154:31–36.

Stokes, P.E. A primary care perspective on the management of acute and long-term depression. *J. Clin. Psychiatry* 1993; 54(supplement 8):74–84.

Thase, M.E. Relapse and recurrence in unipolar major depression: short-term and long-term approaches. *J. Clin. Psychiatry* 1990; 51(supplement 6):51–57.

Antidepressant Discontinuation

Barr, L.C., Goodman, W.K., and Price, L.H. Physical symptoms associated with paroxetine discontinuation. *Am. J. Psychiatry* 1994; 151:289.

Ceccherini-Nelli, A., Bardellini, L., Cur, A., et al. Antidepressant withdrawal: prospective findings. *Am. J. Psychiatry* 1993; 150:165.

Coupland, N.J., Bell, C.J., and Potokar, J.P. Serotonin reuptake inhibitor withdrawal. *J. Clin. Psychopharmacol.* 1996; 16:356–362.

Debattista, C., and Schatzberg, A. Physical symptoms associated with paroxetine withdrawal. *Am. J. Psychiatry* 1995; 152:1235–1236.

Dilsaver, S.C. Antidepressant withdrawal syndromes: phenomenology and pathophysiology. *Acta Psychiatr. Scand.* 1989; 79:113–117.

Dilsaver, S.C., and Greden, J.F. Antidepressant withdrawal phenomenon: a review. *Biol. Psychiatry* 1984; 19:237–256.

Fava, G.A., and Grandi, J. Withdrawal syndromes after paroxetine and sertraline discontinuation. *J. Clin. Psychopharmacol.* 1995; 15:374–375.

Frost, L., and Lal, S. Shock-like sensations after discontinuation of selective serotonin reuptake inhibitors. *Am. J. Psychiatry* 1995; 152:810.

Haddad, P. Newer antidepressants and the discontinuation syndrome. *J. Clin. Psychiatry* 1997; 58(supplement 7):17–22.

Keuthen, M.J., Cyr, P., Riccardi, J., et al. Medication withdrawal symptoms in obsessive-compulsive disorder patients treated with paroxetine. *J. Clin. Psychopharmacol.* 1994; 14:206–207.

Lejoyeux, M., and Ades, J. Antidepressant discontinuation: a review of the literature. *J. Clin. Psychiatry* 1997; 58(supplement 7):11–16.

Louie, A.K., Lannon, R.A., and Agari, L.J. Withdrawal reaction after sertraline discontinuation. *Am. J. Psychiatry* 1994; 151:450–451.

Pyke, R.E. Paroxetine withdrawal syndrome. *Am. J. Psychiatry* 1995; 152:149–150.

Thompson, C (chairperson). Discontinuation of antidepressant therapy: emerging complications and their relevance. *J. Clin. Psychiatry* 1998; 59:541–548.

Zajecka, J., Tracy, K.A., and Mitchell, S. Discontinuation symptoms after treatment with serotonin reuptake inhibitors: a literature review. *J. Clin. Psychiatry* 1997; 58:291–297.

Unilateral Dose Adjustments/Compliance

Basco, M.R., and Rush, A.J. Compliance with pharmacotherapy in mood disorders. *Psychiatric Annals* 1995; 25:269–279.

Blackwell, B. Antidepressant drugs: side effects and compliance. *J. Clin. Psychiatry* 1982; 43:14–18.

Cochran, S.D. Preventing medical noncompliance in the outpatient treatment of bipolar affective disorders. *J. Consult. Clin. Psychology* 1984; 52:873–878.

Demyttenaere, K. Compliance during treatment with antidepressants. *J. Affect. Disord.* 1997; 43:27–39.

Fawcett, J. Compliance: definitions and key issues. *J. Clin. Psychiatry* 1995; 56(supplement 1):4–8.

Frank, E., Kupfer, D.J., and Siegel, L.R. Alliance not compliance: a philosophy of outpatient care. *J. Clin. Psychiatry* 1995; 56(supplement 1):11–16.

Frank, E., Perel, J.M., Mallinger, A.G., et al. Relationship of pharmacologic compliance to long-term prophylaxis in recurrent depression. *Psychopharmacol. Bull.* 1992; 28:231–235.

Lieberman, J.A. III. Compliance issues in primary care. *J. Clin. Psychiatry* 1996; 57(supplement 7):76–82.

Paykel, E.S. Psychotherapy, medication combinations, and compliance. *J. Clin. Psychiatry* 1995; 56(supplement 1):24–30.

Weiss, M., Gaston, L., Propst, A., et al. The role of the alliance in the pharmacologic treatment of depression. *J. Clin. Psychiatry* 1997; 58:196–204.

Drug-Drug Interactions

Ciraulo, D.A., Shader, R.I., Greenblat, D.J., and Creelman, W. *Drug Interactions in Psychiatry, Second Edition.* Williams & Wilkens, Baltimore, 1995.

DeVane, C.L. Pharmacogenetics and drug metabolism of newer antidepressant agents. *J. Clin. Psychiatry* 1994; 55:38–45.

Ereshefsky, L. Drug interactions of antidepressants. *Psychiatric Annals* 1996; 26:342–350.

Ereshefsky, L., Riesenman, C., Lam, L.W.F. Selective serotonin reuptake inhibitor drug interactions and the cytochrome P450 system. *J. Clin. Psychiatry* 1996; 57:17–25.

Greenblatt, D.J., von Moltke, L.L., Harmatz, J.S., and Shader, R.I. Drug interactions with newer antidepressants: role of human cytochromes P450. *J. Clin. Psychiatry* 1998; 59(supplement 15);19–27.

Harvey, A.T., and Preskorn, S.H. Cytochrome P450 enzymes: interpretation of their interactions with selective serotonin reuptake inhibitors, Part I. *J. Clin. Psychopharmacol.* 1996; 16:273–285.

———. Cytochrome P450 enzymes: interpretation of their interactions with selective serotonin reuptake inhibitors, Part II. *J. Clin. Psychopharmacol.* 1996; 16:345–355.

Jefferson, J.W. Drug and diet interactions: avoiding therapeutic paralysis. *J. Clin. Psychiatry* 1998; 59(supplement 16):31–39.

Ketter, T.A., Flockhart, D.A., Post, R.M., et al. The emerging role of cytochrome P450 3A4 in psychopharmacology. *J. Clin. Psychopharmacol.* 1995; 15:387–398.

Lydiard, R.B., Anton, R.F., and Cunningham, T. Interactions between sertraline and tricyclic antidepressants. *Am. J. Psychiatry* 1993; 150:1125–1126.

Maskall, D.D., and Lam, R.W. Increased plasma concentration of imipramine following augmentation with fluvoxamine. *Am. J. Psychiatry* 1993; 150:1566.

Nemeroff, C.B., DeVane, C.L., and Pollock, B.G. Newer antidepressants and the cytochrome P450 system. *Am. J. Psychiatry* 1996; 153:311–320.

Preskorn, S.H. Pharmacokinetics of antidepressants: why and how they are relevant to treatment. *J. Clin. Psychiatry* 1993; 54:14–34.

Preskorn, S.H., Alderman, J., Chung, M., et al. Pharmacokinetics of desipramine coadministered with sertraline or fluoxetine. *J. Clin. Psychopharmacol.* 1994; 14:90–98.

Reeves, R. Serotonin syndrome produced by paroxetine and low-dose trazodone. *Psychosomatics* 1995; 36:159–160.

Richelson, E. Pharmacokinetic interactions of antidepressants. *J. Clin. Psychiatry* 1998; 59(supplement 10):22–26.

Vaughan, D.A. Interaction of fluoxetine with tricyclic antidepressants. *Am. J. Psychiatry* 1988; 145:1478.

Side Effects

Baldwin, D.S., and Birtwistle, J. The side effect burden associated with drug treatment of panic disorder. *J. Clin Psychiatry* 1998; 59(supplement 8):39–46.

Balon, R. (ed.). *Practical Management of the Side Effects of Psychotropic Drugs.* Marcel Dekker, New York, 1998.

Kane, J.M., and Liberman, J.A. (eds.). *Adverse Effects of Psychotropic Drugs.* Guilford Press, New York, 1992.

McElroy, S. Minimizing and managing antidepressant side effects. *J. Clin. Psychiatry* 1995; 56:49–55.

Nierenberg, A.A., Adler, L.A., Peselow, E., et al. Trazodone for antidepressant-associated insomnia. *Am. J. Psychiatry* 1994; 151:1069–1072.

Nierenberg, A.A., and Cole, J.O. Antidepressant adverse drug reactions. *J. Clin. Psychiatry* 1991; 52(supplement 6):40–47.

Nierenberg, A.A., Delgado, P.L., Saks, B.R., and Sussman, N. Antidepressants and sexual dysfunction: a patient-centered approach. *J. Clin. Psychiatry* 1999; 17(monograph 1).

Piazza, L.A., Markowitz, J.C., Kocsis, J.H., et al. Sexual functioning in chronically depressed patients treated with SSRI antidepressants: a pilot study. *Am. J. Psychiatry* 1997; 154:1757–1759.

Rothschild, A.J. Selective serotonin reuptake inhibitor–induced sexual dysfunction: efficacy of a drug holiday. *Am. J. Psychiatry* 1995; 15:341–346.

Segraves, R.T. Overview of sexual dysfunction complicating the treatment of depression. *J. Clin. Psychiatry* 1992; 10(monograph #2):4–10.

Settle, E.C. Antidepressant drugs: disturbing and potentially dangerous adverse effects. *J. Clin. Psychiatry* 1998; 59(supplement 16):25–30.

———. Antidepressant side effects: issues and options. *J. Clin. Psychiatry* 1992; 10:48–65.

Sternbach, H. The serotonin syndrome. *Am. J. Psychiatry* 1991; 148:705–713.

Sussman, N.E., and Ginsberg, D. Rethinking side effects of the selective serotonin reuptake inhibitors: sexual dysfunction and weight gain. *Psychiatric Annals* 1998; 28:89–97.

Tollefson, G.D. Adverse drug reactions/interactions in maintenance therapy. *J. Clin. Psychiatry* 1993; 54(supplement 8):48–58.

Pregnancy

Altshuler, L.L., Cohen, L., Szuba, M.P., et al. Pharmacologic management of psychiatric illness during pregnancy: dilemmas and guidelines. *Am. J. Psychiatry* 1996; 153:592–606.

Altshuler, L.L., and Hendrick, V.C. Pregnancy and psychotropic medication: changes in blood levels. *J. Clin. Psychopharmacol.* 1996; 16:78–80.

Barki, Z.H.K., Kravitz, H.M., and Berki, T.M. Psychotropic medications in pregnancy. *Psychiatric Annals* 1998; 28:486–500.

Cohen, L.S. Psychotropic drug use in pregnancy. *Hosp. Community Psychiatry* 1989; 40:566–567.

Goldstein, D.J., and Marvel, D.C. Psychotropic drug use during pregnancy. *JAMA* 1993; 270:2177.

Kulin, N.A., Pastuszak, A., Sage, S.R., et al. Pregnancy outcome following maternal use of the new selective serotonin reuptake inhibitors: a prospective controlled multicenter study. *JAMA* 1998; 279:609–610.

Lemberg, R., and Phillips, J. The impact of pregnancy on anorexia nervosa and bulimia. *Int. J. Eat. Disord.* 1989; 8:285–295.

Miller, L.J. Clinical strategies for the use of psychotropic drugs during pregnancy. *Psychiatry Med.* 1991; 9:275–298.

————. Psychiatric medication during pregnancy: understanding and minimizing risks. *Psychiatric Annals* 1994; 24:69–75.

Misri, S., and Sivertz, K. Tricyclic drugs in pregnancy and lactation: a preliminary report. *Int. J. Psychiatry Med.* 1991; 21:157–171.

Mortola, J.F. The use of psychotropic agents in pregnancy and lactation. *Psychiatr. Clin. North Am.* 1989; 12:69–87.

Nulman, I., Rovet, J., Stewart, D.E., et al. Neurodevelopment of children exposed in utero to antidepressant drugs. *N. Engl. J. Med.* 1997; 336:258–262.

Pastuszak, A., Schick-Boschetto, B., Zuber, C., et al. Pregnancy outcome following first-trimester exposure to fluoxetine (Prozac). *JAMA* 1993; 269:2246–2248.

Shader, R.I., and Greenblatt, D.J. More on drugs and pregnancy. Editorial. *J. Clin. Psychopharmacol.* 1995; 15:1–2.

Ware, M.R., and DeVane, C.L. Imipramine treatment of panic disorder during pregnancy. *J. Clin. Psychiatry* 1990; 51:482–484.

Webster, P.A.C. Withdrawal symptoms in neonates associated with maternal antidepressant therapy. *Lancet* 1973; 2:318–319.

Wisner, K.L., Perel, J.M., and Wheeler, S.B. Tricyclic dose requirements across pregnancy. *Am. J. Psychiatry* 1993; 150:1541–1542.

Breast-Feeding

Altshuller, L.L., Burt, V.K., McMullen, M., and Hendrick, V. Breastfeeding and sertraline: a 24-hour analysis. *J. Clin. Psychiatry* 1995; 56:243–245.

Breyer-Pafaff, U., Nill, K., Entenmann, A., and Gaertner, H.J. Secretion of amitriptyline and metabolites into breast milk. *Am. J. Psychiatry* 1995; 152:812–813.

Epperson, C.N., Anderson, G.M., and McDougle, C.J. Sertraline and breast-feeding. *N. Engl. J. Med.* 1997; 336:1189–1190.

Erickson, S.H., Smith, G.H., and Heidrich, F. Tricyclics in breast feeding. *Am. J. Psychiatry* 1979; 136:1483.

Jensvold, M.F., Halbreich, U., and Hamilton, J.A. (eds.). *Psychophar-*

macology in Women. American Psychiatric Press, Washington, DC, 1996.

Mammen, O.K., Perel, J.M., Rudolph, G., et al. Sertraline and norsertraline levels in three breastfed infants. *J. Clin. Psychiatry* 1997; 58:100–103.

Matheson, I., Pande, H., and Alertsen, A.R. Respiratory depression caused by N-desmethyldoxepin in breast milk. *Lancet* 1985; 2:1124.

Nulman, I., Rover, J., Stewart, D.E., et al. Neurodevelopment of children exposed in utero to antidepressant drugs. *N. Engl. J. Med.* 1997; 336:258–262.

Spigset, O., and Hagg, S. Excretion of psychotropic drugs into breast milk: pharmacokinetic overview and therapeutic implications. *CNS Drugs* 1998; 9:111–134.

Stancer, H.C., and Reed, K.L. Desipramine and two-hydroxydesipramine in human breast milk and the nursing infant's serum. *Am. J. Psychiatry* 1986; 143:1595–1600.

Stowe, Z.N., Owens, M.J., Landry, J.C., et al. Sertraline and desmethylsertraline levels in human breast milk and nursing infants. *Am. J. Psychiatry* 1997; 154:1255–1260.

Wisner, K.L., and Perel, J.M. Serum nortriptyline levels in nursing mothers and their infants. *Am. J. Psychiatry* 1991; 148:1234–1236.

————. Nortriptyline treatment of breast-feeding women. *Am. J. Psychiatry* 1996; 153:295.

Wisner, K.L., Perel, J.M., and Blumer, J. Serum sertraline and N-desmethylsertraline levels in breast-feeding mother-infant pairs. *Am. J. Psychiatry* 1998; 155:690–692.

Wisner, K.L., Perel, J.M., and Findling, R.L. Antidepressant treatment during breast-feeding. *Am. J. Psychiatry* 1996; 153:1132–1137.

Wisner, K.L., Perel, J.M., and Foglia, J.P. Serum clomipramine and metabolite levels in four nursing mother-infant pairs. *J. Clin. Psychiatry* 1995; 56:17–20.

Yoshida, K., Smith, B., Craggs, M., and Kumar, R.C. Fluoxetine in breast-milk and developmental outcome of breast-fed infants. *Br. J. Psychiatry* 1998; 172:175–179.

Psychotherapy

Agras, W.S. Nonpharmacological treatments of bulimia nervosa. *J. Clin. Psychiatry* 1991; 52(supplement 10):29–33.

Baxter, L.R., Schwartz, J.M., Bergman, K.S., et al. Caudate glucose metabolic rate changes with both drug and behavior therapy for obsessive-compulsive disorder. *Arch. Gen. Psychiatry* 1992; 49:681–689.

Beardslee, W.R., Salt, P., Versage, E.M., et al. Sustained change in parents receiving interventions for families with depression. *Am. J. Psychiatry* 1997; 154:511–515.

Beck, A.T., Hollon, S.D., Young, J.E., et al. Treatment of depression with cognitive therapy and amitriptyline. *Arch. Gen. Psychiatry* 1985; 42:142–148.

Blackburn, I.M., Bishop, S., Glen, A.I.M., et al. The efficacy of cognitive therapy in depression: a treatment trial using cognitive therapy and pharmacotherapy, each alone and in combination. *Br. J. Psychiatry* 1981; 139:181–189.

Blackburn, I.M., Eunson, K.M., Bishop, S. A two-year naturalistic follow-up of depressed patients treated with cognitive therapy, pharmacotherapy, and a combination of both. *J. Affect. Disord.* 1986; 10:67–75.

Clarkin, J.F., Pilkonis, P.A., and Magruder, K.M. Psychotherapy of depression: implications for reform of the healthcare system. *Arch. Gen. Psychiatry* 1996; 53:717–723.

Conte, H.R., Putchik, R., Wild, K.V., and Karasu, T.B. Combined psychotherapy and pharmacotherapy for depression: a systematic analysis of the evidence. *Arch. Gen. Psychiatry* 1986; 43:471–479.

Covi, L., and Lipman, R.S. Cognitive behavioral group psychotherapy combined with imipramine in major depression. *Psychopharmacol. Bull.* 1987; 23:173–176.

Craske, M.G. Cognitive behavioral treatment of panic. In Frances, A., and Hale, R.E. (eds.). *Annual Review of Psychiatry* 7:121–137. American Psychiatric Press, Washington, DC, 1988.

Dar, R., and Greist, J.H. Behavioral treatment of obsessive-compulsive disorder. *Psychiatr. Clin. North Am.* 1992; 15:885–894.

Dimascio, A., Weissman, M.M., Prusoff, B.A., et al. Differential symptom reduction by drugs and psychotherapy in acute depression. *Arch. Gen. Psychiatry* 1979; 36:1450–1456.

Fairburn, C.G., Jones, R., and Peveler, R.C. Three psychological treatments for bulimia nervosa: a comparative trial. *Arch. Gen. Psychiatry* 1991; 48:463–469.

―――. Psychotherapy and bulimia nervosa: longer-term effects of interpersonal psychotherapy, behavior therapy, and cognitive behavior therapy. *Arch. Gen. Psychiatry* 1993; 50:419–428.

Fava, G.A., Grandi, S., Zielezny, M., et al. Four year outcome of cognitive behavioral treatment of residual symptoms in major depression. *Am. J. Psychiatry* 1996; 153:945–947.

Fava, G.A., Rafanelli, C., Grandi, S., et al. Prevention of recurrent depression with cognitive behavioral therapy. *Arch. Gen. Psychiatry* 1998; 55:816–820.

Foley, S.I., Rounsaville, B.J., and Weissman, M.M. Individual versus conjoint interpersonal psychotherapy for depressed patients with marital disputes. *Int. J. Fam. Psychiatry* 1989; 10:29–42.

Frank, E. Interpersonal psychotherapy as a maintenance treatment for patients with recurrent depression. *Psychotherapy* 1991; 28:259–266.

Friedman, A.S. Interaction of drug therapy–marital therapy in depressed outpatients. *Arch. Gen. Psychiatry* 1975; 32:619–637.

Greist, J.H. An integrated approach to treatment of obsessive-compulsive disorder. *J. Clin. Psychiatry* 1992; 53(supplement 4):38–41.

Heimberg, H.G., Liebowitz, M.R., Hope, D.A., et al. Cognitive behavioral group therapy vs phenelzine therapy for social phobia: 12 week outcome. *Arch. Gen. Psychiatry* 1998; 55:1133–1142.

Hersen, M., Bellack, A.S., Himmelhock, J.M., and Thase, M.E. Effects of social skills training, amitriptyline, and psychotherapy in unipolar depressed women. *Behav. Ther.* 1984; 15:21–40.

Hollon, S.D., DeRuveis, R.J., Wiemer, M.H., et al. Cognitive therapy and pharmacotherapy for depression, singly and in combination. *Arch. Gen. Psychiatry* 1992; 49:774–781.

Hollon, S.D., Shelton, R.C., and Loosen, P.T. Cognitive therapy in relation to pharmacotherapy for depression. *J. Consult. Clin. Psychology* 1991; 59:88–99.

Jacobson, N.S., and Hollon, S.D. Cognitive-behavior therapy versus pharmacotherapy: now that the jury's returned its verdict, it's time to present the rest of the evidence. *J. Consult. Clin. Psychology* 1996; 64:74–80.

Katon, W., Robinson, P., Von Korff, M., et al. A multifaceted intervention to improve treatment of depression in primary care. *Arch. Gen. Psychiatry* 1996; 53:924–932.

Keuthen, N.J., O'Sullivan, R.L., Goodchild, P., et al. Behavior therapy and pharmacotherapy for trichotillomania: choice of treatment, patient acceptance, and long-term outcome. *CNS Spectrums* 1998; 3:72–78.

Klerman, G.L. Treatment of recurrent unipolar major depressive disorder. *Arch. Gen. Psychiatry* 1990; 47:1158–1162.

Klerman, G.L., Dimascio, A., Weissman, M.M., et al. Treatment of depression by drugs and psychotherapy. *Am. J. Psychiatry* 1974; 131:186–191.

Kovacs, M., Rush, A.J., Beck, A.T., and Hollon, S.D. Depressed outpatients treated with cognitive therapy or pharmacotherapy: a one-year follow-up. *Arch. Gen. Psychiatry* 1981; 38:33–41.

Markowitz, J.C. *Interpersonal Psychotherapy for Dysthymic Disorder*. American Psychiatric Press, Washington, DC, 1998.

———. Psychotherapy of dysthymia. *Am. J. Psychiatry* 1994; 55:1114–1121.

Marks, I.M. Behavioral treatment of social phobia. *Psychopharmacol. Bull.* 1985; 21:615–618.

———. Advances in behavioral-cognitive therapy of social phobia. *J. Clin. Psychiatry* 1995; 56(supplement 5):25–31.

Michels, M. Psychotherapeutic approaches to the treatment of anxiety and depressive disorders. *J. Clin. Psychiatry* 1997; 58(supplement 13):30–32.

Osgood-Hynes, D.J., Greist, J.H., Marks, I.M., et al. Self-administered psychotherapy for depression using a telephone-accessed computer system plus booklets: an open U.S.-U.K. study. *J. Clin. Psychiatry* 1998; 59:358–365.

Persons, J.B. Indications for psychotherapy in the treatment of depression. *Psychiatric Annals* 1998; 28:80–83.

Persons, J.B., Thase, M.E., and Crits-Cristoph, P. The role of psychotherapy in the treatment of depression: review of two practice guidelines. *Arch. Gen. Psychiatry* 1996; 53:283–290.

Reynolds, C.F., Frank, E., Houck, P.R., et al. Which elderly patients with remitted depression remain well with continued interpersonal psychotherapy after discontinuation of antidepressant medication? *Am. J. Psychiatry* 1997; 154:958–962.

Reynolds, C.F., Frank, E., Perel, J.M., et al. Nortriptyline and interpersonal psychotherapy as maintenance therapies for recurrent major depression. *JAMA* 1999; 281:39–45.

Reynolds, C.F., Miller, M.D., Pasternak, R.E., et al. Treatment of bereavement-related major depressive episodes in later life: a controlled study of acute and continuation treatment with nortriptyline and interpersonal psychotherapy. *Am. J. Psychiatry* 1999; 156:202–207.

Rothbaum, B.O. The behavioral treatment of trichotillomania. *Behav. Psychotherapy* 1992; 20:85–89.

Rush, A.J. (ed.). *Short-term Psychotherapies for Depression*. Guilford Press, New York, 1982.

Sotsky, S.M., Glass, D.R., Shea, M.T., et al. Patient predictors of response to psychotherapy or pharmacotherapy: findings in the NIMH Treatment of Depression Collaborative Research Program. *Am. J. Psychiatry* 1991; 148:997–1008.

Sperry, L. *Psychopharmacology and Psychotherapy: Strategies for Maximizing Treatment Outcome*. Brunner/Mazel, New York, 1995.

Thase, M.E., Dube, S., Bowler, K., et al. Hypothalamic-pituitary-adrenocortical activity and response to cognitive behavior therapy in unmedicated, hospitalized depressed patients. *Am. J. Psychiatry* 1996; 153:886–891.

Thase, M.E., Greenhouse, J.B., Frank, E., et al. Treatment of major depression with psychotherapy or psychotherapy-pharmacotherapy combinations. *Arch. Gen. Psychiatry* 1997; 54:1009–1015.

Walsh, B.T., Wilson, G.T., Loeb, K.L., et al. Medication and psychotherapy in the treatment of bulimia nervosa. *Am. J. Psychiatry* 1997; 154:523–531.

Weissman, M.M. Psychotherapy in the maintenance treatment of depression. *Br. J. Psychiatry* 1994; 165(supplement 26):42–50.

Weissman, M.M., Klerman, G.L., Prusoff, B.A., et al. Depressed outpatients: results one year after treatment with drugs and/or interpersonal psychotherapy. *Arch. Gen. Psychiatry* 1981; 38:51–55.

Weissman, M.M., and Markowitz, J.C. Interpersonal psychotherapy: current status. *Arch. Gen. Psychiatry* 1994; 51:599–608.

Weissman, M.M., Prusoff, B.A., DiMascio, A., et al. The efficacy of drugs and psychotherapy in the treatment of acute depressive episodes. *Am. J. Psychiatry* 1979; 136:555–558.

Wiborg, I.M., and Dahl, A.A. Does brief dynamic psychotherapy reduce the relapse rate of panic disorder? *Arch. Gen. Psychiatry* 1996; 53:689–694.

Wolfe, B., Maser, J.D. (eds.). *The Treatment of Panic Disorder: A Con-*

sensus Development Conference. American Psychiatric Press, Washington, DC, 1994.

Hope

Abrams, R. *Electroconvulsive Therapy, Second Edition.* Oxford University Press, New York, 1992.

American Psychiatric Association. Task Force on Electroconvulsive Therapy. *The Practice of Electroconvulsive Therapy: Recommendations for Treatment, Training, and Privileging: A Task Force Report of the American Psychiatric Association.* American Psychiatric Press, Washington, DC, 1990.

Aronson, R., Offman, H.J., Joffe, R.T., and Naylor, C.D. Triiodothyronine augmentation in the treatment of refractory depression: a meta-analysis. *Arch. Gen. Psychiatry* 1996; 53:842–848.

Benjamin, J., Levine, J., Fux, M., et al. Double-blind, placebo-controlled, crossover trial of inositol treatment for panic disorder. *Am. J. Psychiatry* 1995; 152:1084–1086.

Black, D.W., Winokur, G., and Nazrallah, A. The treatment of depression: ECT versus antidepressants: a naturalistic evaluation of 1,495 patients. *Compr. Psychiatry* 1987; 28:169–182.

Blier, P., and Bergeron, R. The use of pindolol to potentiate antidepressant medication. *J. Clin. Psychiatry* 1998; 59(supplement 5):16–25.

Bloomstein, J.R., Rummans, T.A., Maruta, T., et al. The use of ECT in pain patients. *Psychosomatics* 1996; 37:374–379.

Brujin, J.A., Moleman, P., Mulder, P.G.H., and van den Broek, W.W. Comparison of 2 treatment strategies for depressed inpatients: imipramine and lithium addition or mirtazapine and lithium addition. *J. Clin. Psychiatry* 1998; 59:657–663.

Buchan, H., Johnstone, E., McPherson, K., et al. Who benefits from electroconvulsive therapy: combined results of the Leicester and Northwick Park trials. *Br. J. Psychiatry* 1992; 160:355–359.

Coffey, C.E. (ed.). *The Clinical Science of Electroconvulsive Therapy.* American Psychiatric Press, Washington, DC, 1993.

Cox, B.J., Direnfeld, D.M., Swinson, R.P., et al. Suicide ideation and suicide attempts in panic disorder and social phobia. *Am. J. Psychiatry* 1994; 151:882–887.

Dietrich, D.E., and Emrich, H.M. The use of anticonvulsants to augment antidepressant medication. *J. Clin. Psychiatry* 1998; 59(supplement 5):51–59.

Extein, I.L. (ed.). *Treatment of Tricyclic-Resistant Depression*. American Psychiatric Press, Washington, DC, 1989.

Fava, M., Rosenbaum, J.F., McGrath, P.J., et al. Lithium and tricyclic augmentation of fluoxetine treatment for resistant major depression: a double-blind, controlled study. *Am. J. Psychiatry* 1994; 151:1372–1374.

Fawcett, J. The morbidity and mortality of clinical depression. Special issue: affective disorders: current and future prospectives. *Internat. Clin. Psychopharmacol.* 1993; 8:217–220.

Fawcett, J., Clark, D.C., and Busch, K.A. Assessing and treating the patient at risk for suicide. *Psychiatric Annals* 1993; 23:254–255.

Fernandez, F., Adams, F., Holmes, V.F., et al. Methylphenidate for depressive disorders in cancer patients: an alternative to standard antidepressants. *Psychosomatics* 1987; 28:455–461.

Fink, M. *Convulsive Therapy: Theory and Practice*. Raven Press, New York, 1979.

Fux, M., Levine, J., Aviv, A., and Belmaker, R.H. Inositol treatment of obsessive-compulsive disorder. *Am. J. Psychiatry* 1996; 153:1219–1221.

Gangadhar, B.N., Dapur, R.L., and Kalyanasunduram, S. Comparison of ECT with imipramine in endogenous depression: a double-blind study. *Br. J. Psychiatry* 1982; 141:367–371.

Goodman, W.K., Ward, H.E., and Murphy, T.K. Biologic approaches to treatment-refractory obsessive-compulsive disorder. *Psychiatric Annals* 1998; 28:641–650.

Goodwin, F.K., Prange, A.J., Post, R.M., et al. Potentiation of antidepressant effects by L-triiodothyronine in tricyclic non-responders. *Am. J. Psychiatry* 1982; 139:34–38.

Heninger, G.R., Charney, D.S., and Sternberg, D.E. Lithium carbonate augmentation of antidepressant treatment: an effective prescription for treatment-refractory depression. *Arch. Gen. Psychiatry* 1983; 40:1335–1342.

Hollander, E., and Cohen, L.J. The assessment and treatment of refractory anxiety. *J. Clin. Psychiatry* 1994; 55(supplement 2):27–31.

Jefferson, J.J., Akiskal, H.S., Nierenberg, A.A., et al. Management of patients who are non-responders to, or non-tolerators of, initial antidepressant therapy. *J. Clin. Psychiatry* 1992; 10(monograph 1).

Joffe, R.T. The use of thyroid supplements to augment antidepressant medication. *J. Clin. Psychiatry* 1998; 59(supplement 5):26–31.

Joffe, R.T., Singer, W., Levitt, A.J., et al. A placebo-controlled comparison of lithium and triiodothyronine augmentation of tricyclic antidepressants in unipolar refractory depression. *Arch. Gen. Psychiatry* 1993; 50:387–393.

Kindler, S., Shapira, B., Hadjez, J., et al. Factors influencing response to bilateral electroconvulsive therapy in major depression. *Convulsive Therapy* 1991; 7:245–254.

Klein, E., Kreinin, I., Chistyakov, A., et al. Therapeutic efficacy of right prefrontal slow repetitive transcranial magnetic stimulation in major depression. *Arch. Gen. Psychiatry* 1999; 56:315–320.

Kramer, M.S., Cutler, N., Feigner, J., et al. Distinct mechanism for antidepressant activity by blockade of central substance P receptors. *Science* 1998; 281:1640–1645.

Kroessler, D., and Fogel, B.S. Electroconvulsive therapy for major depression in the oldest old. *Am. J. Geriatric Psychiatry* 1993; 1:30–37.

Masand, P., Pickett, P., and Murray, G.B. Psychostimulants for secondary depression in medical illness. *Psychosomatics* 1991; 32:201–208.

Murphy, B.E., Dhar, V., Ghardirian, A.M., et al. Response to steroid suppression in major depression resistant to antidepressant therapy. *J. Clin. Psychopharmacol.* 1991; 11:121–126.

Nelson, J.C. Augmentation strategies with serotonergic-noradrenergic combinations. *J. Clin. Psychiatry* 1998; 59(supplement 5):65–69.

———. Combined drug treatment strategies for major depression. *Psychiatric Annals* 1998; 28:197–203.

———. Overcoming treatment resistance in depression. *J. Clin. Psychiatry* 1998; 59(supplement 16):13–19.

Nelson, J.C., and Mazure, C.M. Lithium augmentation in psychotic depression refractory to combined drug treatment. *Am. J. Psychiatry* 1986; 143:363–366.

Nemeroff, C.B. Augmentation regimens for depression. *J. Clin. Psychiatry* 1991; 52:21–27.

Nierenberg, A.A. What next? A review of pharmacologic strategies for treatment-resistant depression. *Psychopharmacol. Bull.* 1990; 26:429–460.

Nierenberg, A.A., Dougherty, D., and Rosenbaum, J. Dopaminergic agents and stimulants as antidepressant augmentation strategies. *J. Clin. Psychiatry* 1998; 59(supplement 5):61–64.

Nolen, W.A., Zohar, J., Roose, S.P., and Amsterdam, J.D. (eds.). *Refractory Depression: Current Strategies and Future Directions.* John Wiley & Sons, Chichester, England, 1994.

Olin, J., and Masand, P. Psychostimulants for depression in hospitalized cancer patients. *Psychosomatics* 1996; 37:57–62.

Oquendo, M.A., Malone, K.M., Ellis, S.P., et al. Inadequacy of antidepressant treatment for patients with major depression who are at risk for suicidal behavior. *Am. J. Psychiatry* 1999; 156:190–194.

O'Reardon, J.P., Amsterdam, J.P. Treatment-resistant depression: progress and limitations. *Psychiatric Annals* 1998; 28:633–641.

Perez, V., Gilberte, I., Faries, D., et al. Randomized, double-blind, placebo-controlled trial of pindolol in combination with fluoxetine antidepressant treatment. *Lancet* 1997; 349:1594–1597.

Petrides, G. Continuation ECT: a review. *Psychiatric Annals* 1998; 28:517–523.

Phillips, K.A., and Nierenberg, A.A. The assessment and treatment of refractory depression. *J. Clin. Psychiatry* 1994; 55(supplement Z):20–26.

Pigott, T.A., Pato, M.T., L'Heureaux, F., et al. A controlled comparison of adjuvant lithium carbonate or thyroid hormone in clomipramine-treated patients with obsessive-compulsive disorder. *J. Clin. Psychopharmacol.* 1991; 11:242–248.

Potter, W.Z., and Manjis, H.K. Refractory depression: is there a next step? *Psychiatric Annals* 1994; 24:505–507.

Prange, A., Wilson, I.C., and Rabon, A.M. Enhancement of imipramine antidepressant activity by thyroid. *Am. J. Psychiatry* 1969; 126:457–469.

Roemer, R.A., Dubin, D.W.R., Joffe, R., et al. An efficacy study of single versus double-seizure induction with ECT in major depression. *J. Clin. Psychiatry* 1990; 51:473–478.

Rouillon, F., and Gorwood, P. The use of lithium to augment antidepressant medication. *J. Clin. Psychiatry* 1998; 59(supplement 5):32–41.

Satel, S.L., and Nelson, J.C. Stimulants in the treatment of depression: a critical overview. *J. Clin. Psychiatry* 1989; 50:241–249.

Schaff, M.R., Fawcett, J., and Zajecka, J.M. Divalproex sodium in the treatment of refractory affective disorders. *J. Clin. Psychiatry* 1993; 54:380–384.

Schopf, S., Baumann, P., LeMarchand, T., et al. Treatment of endogenous depressions resistant to tricyclic antidepressant or related drugs by lithium addition. *Pharmacopsychiatry* 1984; 22:183–187.

Shelton, R.C. Treatment options for refractory depression. *J. Clin. Psychiatry* 1999; 60(supplement 4):57–63.

———. Mood-stabilizing drugs in depression. *J. Clin. Psychiatry* 1999; 60(supplement 5):37–46.

Sobin, C., Prudic, J., Devanand, P., et al. Who responds to electroconvulsive therapy? A comparison of effective and ineffective forms of treatment. *Br. J. Psychiatry* 1996; 169:322–328.

Stoudemire, A. Expanding psychopharmacologic treatment options for the depressed medical patient. *Psychosomatics* 1995; 36:519–526.

Sussman, N. Anxiolytic antidepressant augmentation. *J. Clin. Psychiatry* 1998; 59(supplement 5):42–50.

Sussman, N., Joffe, R.T. Introduction: augmentation of antidepressant medication. *J. Clin. Psychiatry* 1998; 59(supplement 5): 3–4.

———. Antidepressant augmentation: conclusions and recommendations. *J. Clin. Psychiatry* 1998; 59(supplement 5):70–73.

Thase, M.E., Howland, R.H., and Friedman, E.S. Treating antidepressant nonresponders with augmentation strategies: an overview. *J. Clin. Psychiatry* 1998; 59(supplement 5):5–15.

Thase, M.E., Kupfer, D.J., Frank, E., et al. Treatment of imipramine-resistant recurrent depression, II: an open clinical trial of lithium augmentation. *J. Clin. Psychiatry* 1989; 50:413–417.

Thase, M.E., and Rush, A.J. When at first you don't succeed: sequential strategies for antidepressant nonresponders. *J. Clin. Psychiatry* 1997; 58(supplement 13):23–29.

Tiffon, L., Coplan, J.D., Papp, L.A., et al. Augmentation strategies with tricyclic or fluoxetine in seven partially responsive panic disorder patients. *J. Clin. Psychiatry* 1994; 55:66–69.

Wheatley, D. Potentiation of amitriptyline by thyroid hormones. *Arch. Gen. Psychiatry* 1972; 26:229–233.

Wilson, I.C., Prange, A.J., McClane, T.K., et al. Thyroid-hormone enhancement of imipramine in non-retarded depressions. *N. Engl. J. Med.* 1979; 282:1063–1067.

Young, M.A., Fogg, L.F., Scheftner, W.A., and Fawcett, J.A. Interactions of risk factors in predicting suicide. *Am. J. Psychiatry* 1994; 151:434–435.

Zajecka, J.M., Jeffries, H., and Fawcett, J. The efficacy of fluoxetine combined with a heterocyclic antidepressant in treatment-resistant depression: a retrospective analysis. *J. Clin. Psychiatry* 1995; 56:338–343.

Index

social phobia
  medications for, 26, 207
  overview of, 34
  resources on, 231–32
spirituality, 108
SSRI (selective serotonin
  reuptake inhibitor)
  antidepressants, 18, 19
stealing, compulsive, 31, 121–
  22, 239
stopping antidepressant
  medication, 146–47, 259–
  60
stress
  as cause of disorder, 180
  staying on medication in
  times of, 140–41
"strong" antidepressant, 48
substance use
  informing doctor of, 91–96
  mixing with antidepressant
  use, 154–58
  resources on, 253–55
suicide
  antidepressants and, 55–56
  frequency of, 24
  hopelessness and, 198, 200–1
  resources on, 245–46
surgery and medication, 169–
  70
Surmontil (trimipramine), 207
symptom-focused approach to
  evaluation by doctor, 62,
  64–65, 67
symptoms
  as cause of disorder, 182
  chronological history of, 77–
  83
  fluctuations in, 131–35

genetic factors in, 83–86
nonpharmacological
  techniques to improve,
  107–8
relapses and recurrences of,
  192–93, 195–96
See also target symptoms
synapse, 15–16

tapering off medication, 146–
  47
target dose of medication, 119–
  20
target symptoms
  identifying and clarifying,
  62, 64–65, 109
  prioritizing, 67
therapeutic alliance with
  doctor, 59–60, 99–100,
  200
therapeutic blood level of
  medicine, 128–29
therapy
  advantages of, 186–88
  combining medication with,
  47, 107, 186–88
  discontinuing, 141
  historical preference for, 43
  resources on, 266–70
Thorazine, 14, 18
timing of dose of medication,
  123–27
Tofranil (imipramine), 14, 17,
  18, 207
tolerance to drugs, 52
total daily dose of medication,
  119, 126